Am I
My Own
Miracle?

AM I
MY OWN
MIRACLE?

Journey to Recovery

ELAINE ROSENDORF

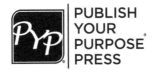

PUBLISH
YOUR
PURPOSE
PRESS

For permission requests, write to the publisher, addressed "Attention: Permissions Coordinator," at the address below.

Publish Your Purpose Press
141 Weston Street, #155
Hartford, CT, 06141

The opinions expressed by the Author are not necessarily those held by Publish Your Purpose Press.

Ordering Information: Quantity sales and special discounts are available on quantity purchases by corporations, associations, and others. For details, contact the author at elaine@amberworldwide.com.

Edited by: Fern Pessin, Caroline Davis
Typeset by: Medlar Publishing Solutions Pvt Ltd., India

Printed in the United States of America.
ISBN: 978-1-951591-63-2 (paperback)
ISBN: 978-1-951591-64-9 (ebook)

Library of Congress Control Number: 2021900805

First edition, April 2021.

The information contained within this book is strictly for informational purposes. The material may include information, products, or services by third parties. As such, the Author and Publisher do not assume responsibility or liability for any third-party material or opinions. The publisher is not responsible for websites (or their content) that are not owned by the publisher. Readers are advised to do their own due diligence when it comes to making decisions.

The mission of Publish Your Purpose Press is to discover and publish authors who are striving to make a difference in the world. We give marginalized voices power and a stage to share their stories, speak their truth, and impact their communities. Do you have a book idea you would like us to consider publishing? Please visit PublishYourPurposePress.com for more information.

To
my husband, Keith,
who promised to love me forever,
and proved forever does exist.

ACKNOWLEDGMENT

My thanks

To Dr. S Robert Rozbruch, who, unlike all the king's horses and all the king's men, did put me back together again.

To all the other doctors, nurses, physical therapists, and aides whose hands helped me to heal.

To the members of the Writers Studio of the Delray Beach Public Library who encouraged and motivated me "to just keep writing."

To Fern Pessin, manuscript strategist, who helped me to clarify my thoughts and design the front and back covers.

To Publish Your Purpose Press and everyone involved in the production and marketing of my book.

CONTENTS

FOREWORD

I am an orthopedic surgeon specializing in limb reconstruction. Elaine was in a terrible car accident in which she sustained a femur fracture. After treatment elsewhere, we could see the bone was not healing properly thereby affecting her mobility, which is what brought her to me.

Accompanied by her loving husband Keith, Elaine made an immediate strong impression on me. Stylish, energetic, and smart describe the seventy year old woman who was determined to get back to the busy and fulfilling life she shared with Keith.

A major surgery was needed to heal Elaine and regain her quality of life. I performed a repair of the femur nonunion with revision of hardware and bone grafting.

Recovery certainly has much to do with the extent of trauma and the quality of treatment, but equally important is the mental state and attitude of the patient. Elaine's optimistic attitude, positive energy, and determination despite an initial setback was inspiring and so important in her recovery. She had a purpose, and it was to return to the great life she had before the accident.

I really enjoyed treating the remarkable Elaine and getting to know her. I encouraged her to write about her journey of recovery. Elaine has something important to share with others facing adversity. This book is sure to inspire and give strength and purpose to those who read it.

S. Robert Rozbruch, MD

Attending Orthopaedic Surgeon | Hospital for Special Surgery;
Chief | Limb Lengthening and Complex Reconstruction Service (LLCRS);
Director | Limb Salvage and Amputation Reconstruction Center (LSARC);
Professor of Clinical Orthopaedic Surgery;
Weill Cornell Medicine, Cornell University

PREFACE

At seventy years old, you almost feel like you can breathe a sigh of relief. You've gotten through the challenges of school, finding a partner, building a career (or something fulfilling to occupy your time and earn income), raising children, creating a home, cultivating a group of truly special and caring friends, becoming comfortable in your relationship with God/religion (whatever that is or isn't) and basically having it all together. You know your aging body is going to start bringing new adventures, but the rest of it should be well in hand, right? Well, as the Yiddish expression goes, "We make plans and god laughs!"

At seventy years old, two minutes changed my entire life. Everything that was routine, the lifestyle I was living, and all my life's priorities were upended, and I basically had to reboot. This book reflects back on what happened and the impact this recovery rollercoaster had on who I am today.

My surgeon asked me to write this book because my recovery was, in his words, miraculous. He felt that my belief that I would recover and return to my life was what made everyone else believe in me and work to help me get where I was determined to be. He said my journey to recovery would inspire older people facing crisis not to resign themselves to what appeared to be their fate.

Before writing this book, I did some internet research to try to remember all the exercises I did in the rehab center. My heart raced, and my skin crawled with goose bumps as I realized why everyone at the Hospital for Special Surgery referred to me as "the miracle." The statistics for broken femurs, never mind *shattered* femurs, were not optimistic for older people. The aftermath of infection, permanent disability, as well as the mortality rate was much higher than in younger patients. It's a good thing I didn't look this up while I was still recovering, or I may have been tempted to give up.

My memories of my experience from start to finish are relatively clear, except for several black holes that have never filled in. I share my story as I experienced it and with whatever memories I have been able to excavate from my mind. Some of the names have been deliberately changed, and others I cannot remember, so I've made substitutions.

As I write this, it is now eight years later. I am retired, living on my own, and quite literally standing on my own two feet. I encourage you to maximize your mind, body, and spirit; to live the life you want to live and be the person you want to be. No matter the challenges, DON'T QUIT. It is only when you harness your thought processes and brain that you realize how *powerful* you are! You can overcome anything!

Wishing you all the best,
Elaine

CHAPTER 1

THE ACCIDENT—APRIL 24, 2012

"What the fuck was that?" The words tumbled out of my mouth, rapid fire, tinged with annoyance and anger, in an accusatory tone directed at my husband. I had let the soothing, rocking motion of the car lull me into a nap as we were driving home from the dentist on a spectacular New York spring day. The sun was bright in the sky. Flowers, bushes, and trees were blooming. The air, permeated with all the combined fragrances, was beautiful, not offensive to the senses. As my eyes opened, I recognized what *that* was. It was the sound of metal caving in on itself. Anyone who has ever heard that sound would never forget it; it would be forever etched in the brain.

My mind now recalls it all as a slide show. My newly opened, sleepy eyes took in everything around me. Our car, a Mitsubishi SUV, was off the ground, rotating. Everything in the car was spinning through the air. Papers, a mini umbrella, business files, tossed about in a tornado-like funnel. To write this paragraph takes longer than the actual duration of the event, but the recollection is as vivid today, all these years later, as when it was just happening.

The car made two complete rotations before slamming onto the ground with an enormous thud and a terrific vibration. My senses absorbed the sound of a pop and whoosh, the feeling of sudden pressure as the airbag pushing me back against the seat. My brain was still sorting images of contents flying around in a circle—until, as the car ceased rotating, all the spinning items slowed and came to rest wherever.

My eyes searched for my husband. He was not in the car. The driver's door was open. On my side of the car, the air bag had me crushed against the seat back. I screamed for Keith. I moved my head slowly and noticed the door on my side was gone. I could not see past the air bag to the outside. There was no response from Keith. I called again. The safety glass from the windshield and the windows had crystallized and shimmered over everything like tiny diamonds in the sunlight.

My left knee was married to the dashboard. I could feel the pressure. My left foot had no feeling. I could not move it, not even a little. I could not see over the airbag to check my foot.

The airbag held me firmly in place. I could not move anything else, so I started to move my hands. I could feel both hands, but the ring finger and pinky at the end of my right hand had very little feeling. I moved my left hand to my left leg. My leg didn't move. It didn't feel like it had fallen asleep—more that it was no longer a part of me.

My right hand could feel the car seat, and then my pants, and then my right leg. As I moved my hands upward, I could feel a bump. Not rounded, but kind of angular. I knew then that the bone was broken. *Strange*, I thought. I could feel that the area was dry.

No blood? So maybe it wasn't the bone. I was not in any pain, just the pressure from the airbag.

And still no husband. I worried about what had become of Keith. Was he alive? Was he hurt? Did he know that I was still in the car?

I questioned myself… Was I alive or dead? They say that when you die, you can see yourself as the soul leaves the body. From what I had read about out-of-body experiences, you viewed yourself from above. Here I was, viewing everything the same way I always had, so what did that mean?

I heard a voice shouting. I looked to the right. I saw a man in a gray suit standing on the sidewalk with a cell phone in his hand, yelling to me that he had called 911 and that the police and fire department were on the way.

A woman came close to the car on my side. I asked her, "Have you seen my husband? He was driving. Is he okay? Alive? Hurt?"

"Not to worry, dear," she responded. "Your husband was some-how able to get out of the car. He is pretty banged up, but he can talk, and I think he must be in shock because a lot of what he's say-ing doesn't make any sense. He keeps asking for his glasses. He says he cannot see. And he's asking for you."

"Can you see my purse?" I asked. "I need my purse! I have to have it."

"Yes, dear. Keep calm. Help is on the way. Your purse is in the driver's seat. It's not open. It's not damaged."

"I need my cell phone. I have to call him. He needs to hear my voice," I pleaded.

"Try to stay calm," she repeated. "Help is on the way. I'll go over to your husband and tell him I have spoken to you and that you are alive. And I'll see if he has his cell phone. Who do you want called?"

The man in the gray suit walked a little closer to the car. He assured me that the fire department had been called and was coming. Then he turned and left.

I knew my contact lenses were still in my eyes because I could see. Without them, I realized, everything would have been blurred. I kept trying to locate Keith. Where was he?

A thought crossed my mind that it was strange that nothing hurt. And then I heard a voice behind me.

"My name is John. I am an EMT. I am here to help you. I want you to bring your hands under the airbag and cross them in front of your chest. I will grab hold of your hands with my hands. I don't want you to move. Not any part of your body except your hands. Okay? Understand? I will not leave you until the fire department arrives."

"Okay," I said. The airbag seemed less tight, and I was able to do what John asked of me. "Why are you here exactly? Have the police asked you to come?"

"I was in my pickup on my way home from work and saw the result of the accident. Didn't see the actual accident, but I came over to see if I could help. The police are here," John said.

I interrupted. "My husband?"

"An ambulance has arrived, and I assume it'll be taking him to the hospital, same one you'll be going to. There's a trauma hospital not too far away. Due to shock, he needs to be kept quiet. No one will be sure about the extent of his injuries until he is examined. I saw him. He knows you are alive, and he knows that the trauma hospital has dispatched a helicopter. He knows that the fire department is on the way."

"Can he come here? Can he walk? I need to see him!" I pleaded.

"No. I don't think so." He said quite calmly, his words soothing me with their reassuring tone. "I can see they are putting him in the ambulance now. They are checking him out. Don't worry. It is critical to get you both examined as soon as possible. I will stay here with you until the fire department comes and until you are free."

"Why the fire department?" I asked.

"They will have the tools to cut you out of the car. They have the jaws of life." Terrifying images started playing in my head.

CHAPTER 2

UNTANGLING

I don't remember all of what John and I spoke about. He said it was important for us to keep the conversation going. I don't think we discussed what caused the accident because I was asleep when it happened.

"Do you have children?" he asked.

"Two," I replied. "Sons."

"How old?"

"Forty-seven and forty-five."

"Do they live close by?"

"One in Westchester, one in Miami."

"Are they married or single? Kids?" he prompted.

"Married. My older son has three; the younger, one."

And this was how it went on. Looking back, I realized he never asked me my name or if I lived around there. He didn't ask about what I did for a living or anything about my husband. He didn't ask where we were going or anything else about me actually. He never asked if he could call my kids (or anyone else) for me. He just kept the conversation going with innocuous questions that I freely answered. Other than telling me his name was John, he never mentioned anything about himself either.

I wanted to ask him to pull down the visor in front of me so I could see what my face looked like in the visor mirror. There were several parts of my face, especially the cheeks, that seemed to crackle as I spoke. *Must be glass*, I thought. Glass was all over the place. Everywhere I looked, there were a thousand shards. I thought better of asking for the mirror view. Did I really want to see the *American Horror Story* up front and up close?

My leg began to throb a bit. Time had no definitive beginning or end.

Where's Keith? Where's my husband? Where is he? Why isn't he here? was running through my mind on a loop. I asked the questions aloud. John reminded me that Keith had already been taken to the hospital and I would be able to see him there.

"Stay calm," he said. "I'm your new friend." His voice was so soft and kind, and it reassured me.

I finally heard sirens and bells. How much time had passed? I could see the firetruck coming down the road. It veered slightly to the right to avoid a fallen lamppost before coming to a stop.

A man in a military-style cap appeared at the driver's door. He wasn't wearing a fireman's helmet. I was momentarily confused. He introduced himself as Captain Bowski of the Long Beach Fire Department. He stated that he was in charge of a specialized department, and that his squad would be cutting away the twisted and bent metal so they could get me out of the car. He asked if I had any pain.

I said, "No. Not much. Just some throbbing in my leg."

He asked questions and I answered. "What's your name? Where do you live? Was anyone else in the car?" And then he said, "The police notified me about the accident, your husband, and you."

Mangled would be the best word to describe the right side of the car. It was the first time I had actually paid attention to its condition. The edge of a light pole was hanging on the outside of the car. The fender was now a part of the hood. And the hood? Well, it didn't seem to fit onto the crunched-up car anymore!

I asked the captain, "Do you see my handbag on the seat? A lady said it was right there; I need to be sure I have it. I need to hold on to it. It has my wallet and phone. I need to call my husband and tell him I am okay. I AM okay, right?"

"Don't worry, young woman," he replied with a nice smile. "I see it. It will go with you to the hospital."

Then the captain explained what I was about to hear. "My squad will be making a lot of noise as they cut you out of this wreckage. There is no other way to get you out. Once we can see all of you, we will assess how to move you. The loud whirring you're hearing is a helicopter dispatched from NUMC [Nassau University Medical Center]. You'll be put on a stretcher with wheels that will be lifted into the helicopter, and you'll be flown to the hospital."

"Young woman?" I scoffed. "You need new glasses! I'm old enough to be your grandmother! I'm seventy years old!"

While laughing at my remarks, he added, "Before I can give you more info, I need to get a handle on your pulse. I can do this by putting my hand on your neck, as the airbag has completely enveloped you." And as he reached over, he added with a grin, "You look like you've been eaten by a giant marshmallow."

That made me laugh, but it hurt. I kept smiling as I imagined the graphic image of me being eaten by a marshmallow.

As I looked to my right, I could see the tops of the helmets of two firemen and hear the crunching of metal as they worked on the car.

"Where's my husband?" I asked again.

The captain replied, "He has been taken by ambulance to NUMC. I have this information directly from the police officers. He's already in the ER."

"Now," he said, "I want you to concentrate on what I'm going to tell you. Once you are free, you'll be lifted onto a stretcher, and you'll be strapped in. Your head will be positioned so you cannot move it. Do not be scared. We need to keep you as immobile as possible to avoid adding to the injuries you have sustained."

I was suddenly aware that the crunching sound had stopped. I had not heard any more from John. My hands were still criss-crossed, holding onto my body.

"Where's John?" I asked.

"Who?" the captain replied.

"You know, the guy that was sitting behind me."

"What guy?" he asked. "I never saw anyone here. Was he a passenger?"

"No. Only me and my husband were in the car. He came once the car landed. His name was John. He was an EMT. He's been speaking to me. He told me to cross my arms and he was here talking to me a few minutes ago. You haven't seen him?"

"No, lady. I just see you."

I thought about John a lot in the weeks and months that followed the accident. How can you identify someone by a voice? I put ads in the local paper, asking him to contact me. I asked if anyone at the scene of the accident had seen him or his truck. Many weeks of ads, no response.

The guy in the gray suit sent me an email. He wrote that he did not remember seeing any pickup near the car. The lady with the kind face also emailed me the same.

I even offered a reward if anyone could give me information. No response. I tried for a year and then gave up.

I knew later that due to the extent of my injuries, I should have been dead. So, who was John? That question remains unanswered to this date. I definitely felt his hands and heard his voice. Ultimately, I wondered if John was real or if I had been hallucinating? Maybe he was an angel?

CHAPTER 3

HEADING TO THE ER

There are clear memories about the accident that stay with me until today, while other time gaps appear as vast black holes. The individual images that come to me when I close my eyes, click, click, click, pass by like a backyard slide show.

I do not remember exactly how they removed me from the car. I do recall the feeling that somehow the airbag was no longer pushing me into the seat back. Voices drifted in and out, most likely in sync with my level of consciousness. Commentary from the firemen indicated that my left knee was embedded into the dashboard and my left foot and shoe were perpendicular to one another.

The next thing I remember was the attendant in the helicopter giving my vitals to whomever was on the other end of the radio at the hospital. What struck me were the numbers he read off for my blood pressure: 220 over 110. My normal BP was around 110 over 65. Hearing that new number made me realize that I could, well, maybe be dying! Or worse, my mind corrected, living but maybe paralyzed. I still felt no pain.

Panic had not been a word in my vocabulary until that moment, so I cannot relay my exact feelings except that my thoughts turned to all the things I had left undone, and then, to Keith. He had been driving. Guilt feelings, even if I did not die, would most likely occupy his thoughts. How would he handle it?

The hum and vibration of the helicopter stopped as we landed. Suddenly, I felt extreme pain coursing throughout my body. Had they given me a painkiller when they took me up? I thought not, but perhaps they did. This is one of those black holes. The mind is a very strange and wonderful thing.

The attendants that met the helicopter took charge and were running alongside the stretcher as we zoomed down a hallway. I could not turn my immobilized head in any direction, as it was encased in some kind of helmet contraption. I was flat on my back, and the only thing I could see were the ceiling tiles and fluorescent lights passing above me. I felt like I was in one of those medical drama television shows like *Grey's Anatomy*. Whatever made me think of that?

The racing suddenly stopped. I was surrounded by at least five people, asking me tons of questions all at the same time. Only one response came to my mind. "I am in terrible pain!" I screamed. "You need to stop the pain! Give me something!" And I started to shake. Not really shake, more shiver. There wasn't a part of my body that wasn't shivering. I could not remember ever being so cold. A nurse with a kind face leaned over me, smiled, and said they would get me a blanket.

The question assault began again. Over and over they asked, "What is your name? Where do you live? How old are you?"

Two men in surgical masks and black-rimmed glasses came and stood over me. "I am Dr. Bruce Wayne, and this is Dr. Robin

Friedman, and we will be taking care of you. We are here to assess your injuries. We have the report from the helicopter."

What passed through my mind? *Batman and Robin are here to take care of me!?* And then I presumed maybe I was only dreaming.

The nurse with the kind face started narrating each item as she was removing my jewelry. She put my rings, watch, earrings, and the chain around my neck into a plastic bag with my name on it.

Another nurse had a huge pair of scissors and was cutting my jacket off my body. Someone else was removing my shoe, I think. The nurse cautioned the other attendants not to pull the pants but to cut them off instead. She told me that they needed to cut away my clothing to keep movement to a minimum.

The intense cold I felt outweighed the pain or embarrassment. Every part of my body continued to shake and shiver as I was stripped down naked. I repeated my plea to be covered and warmed. I was covered with what felt like a sheet, but it might have been a blanket. Either way, it did not help. I was not moving but still shivering.

The questions started again. "What's your husband's name?" asked the kind-faced nurse.

"Keith. Keith Milliner."

"He has been admitted and is being examined," she assured me. "Your handbag is here, and we will take care of it for you and will give it to your husband along with the jewelry."

Dr. Batman (I could only think of him in this way), said they would be moving me to another table, and they would be washing me with warm water. "It will feel like a shower," he informed, and afterwards they would wrap me in a large bag that would be filled with blowing warm air.

I felt the prick of several needles going into my legs, elevating the pain. What was wrong with these people? Did they not realize how much pain I was already in? I remember screaming, "Oh God, oh God, help me! Help me!" The shivers got worse, and the pain seemed to increase, and then they moved me. The other table was in front of me and a little to the right. At this point, all I kept thinking, begging God, let me die. PLEASE! At least the pain would stop.

During the shift from gurney to table, I caught a glimpse of my leg, which was bent at the knee with the bone protruding. I threw up. I remember that.

Once I was on the other table, they hosed me down with some kind of solution. It was yellow and warm. I remember I just kept screaming.

Dr. Batman stood above me, grabbed my right foot, and gave it a big jerk. Death would have been better!

Through the pain and screams, a part of my brain was preoccupied with John Wayne in a western I had seen, where he did that same maneuver to a man who had fallen off his horse and broken his arm. Later, Keith told me that he could hear me screaming from the other side of the ER.

At this point, maybe I passed out. When I woke up, I wasn't so cold anymore. I recognized warm air blowing on me once I was encased in the bag. I was in a bed, covered by blankets, and both of my legs were covered. They must have been wrapped because they appeared to be twice as large as normal and I could not move them.

My hands were free, and I lifted them to my face. I couldn't feel the touch of my fingers on my face, but my fingertips explored a series of tapes on the skin. I was awash with relief as the pain was nearly gone from my body, except for the heaviness in my chest area. I put my hands under the gown and felt what seemed to be ice bags.

My eyes closed as I tried to come to grips with what was happening to me. After a few minutes, a nurse came by. "How are you feeling, my dear?" she asked solicitously. "Are you in any pain and if so, where?" I told her about my chest. "Well, you are badly bruised from the airbag (which undoubtedly saved your life). I'm told that the car you were in was scattered over most of the roadway. But you are in good hands here. Our hospital is the only trauma hospital in Nassau County and the only one with a helicopter. We have the best of the best here, to treat all kinds of injuries."

"What kind of injuries do I have?"

"Well, I know that you have a broken right femur, and that you have had stitches on your left knee; a broken left ankle; and you have several contusions, especially on your right arm and chest."

"And my face? I felt it and it has funny patches on it, I think."

"They removed some glass shards, cleaned the wounds, and covered them. There were not too many and from what I know, not too deeply embedded. They will heal and I think no scarring will occur."

"I am thirsty. Can you get me some water please?"

"No, darling," she answered sympathetically. "You are scheduled to go for surgery sometime in the early hours of the morning. We apologize for this, but there is another patient in worse condition than you, and the doctors felt you could stand the wait. The best I can do is give you some swabs that you can put in your mouth."

"What time is it?"

"About 11:00 p.m.," she responded.

"Where's my husband? Is he hurt? Can he come here?"

"Give me his name and I'll see what I can find out."

As she left, Dr. Batman walked in. He said he had done all he could for the present but that I required surgery to stabilize me. Then he asked, "What's your level of pain?"

"About a five, I think."

"We will be giving you some more pain medications by IV in a few minutes, and you may be able to sleep. Try. It will help with the wait."

He continued, "Your husband, I know you have been asking about him. He's been treated mainly for cuts and bruises and is doing okay. I will be back later. Oh, and they will be taking you downstairs as soon as we have the operating room free."

CHAPTER 4

FIRST SURGERY—APRIL 25TH

I awoke in a large, dimly lit room and could hear voices all around me. A nurse was standing over me. She didn't realize I was awake as when I spoke, she looked a little startled. I asked her where I was. She told me I was near the nurse's station closest to the operating room.

"Why?" I wanted to know. "How come I'm not in a regular room?"

"It's easier for the nurses to monitor you from here, before you go in for surgery." She added, "Do you know where you are?"

"Nassau Hospital."

"Do you know why you are here?"

"I was in a car accident. I remember the helicopter, and then the ER, and not too much else. Except I remember screaming, and the cold and the pain. I guess I'm here with you, now. Why am I being operated on?"

"You have bad injuries to both your legs."

"Did they x-ray me? I don't remember anything past the bath they gave me and the incredible pain. I must've passed out. I'm thirsty. Can I have some water please?"

"No. The only thing I can give you is some mouthwash swabs to put under your tongue. No liquids permitted before surgery. Let me get you some swabs."

Before she could leave, I asked, "Do you know where my husband is? Is he okay?"

"I will check on your chart and see if there are notes." Then she winked at me and joked, "Now don't go anywhere; I'll be right back."

"Before you go…" I stopped her again from leaving. "I still have my contacts in my eyes. I need to take them out."

"You need to stay quiet and lying down."

"No! I have hard lenses. I need to sit up. Call a doctor to take them out for me. They should have a little thing that looks like a plunger."

"Sorry," she said. "The ophthalmic department is closed. Let me get you those swabs." And she started to walk away.

To her retreating back I said angrily, "This is a hospital! Nothing should be closed! I need to get these out. What if my eyes get too dry and they are pasted to my eyeballs? You can't tell me there is no one here to help. Sit me up. Now!"

After all the trauma I had gone through—the incredible pain, the unquenched thirst, worrying about my husband and not knowing for sure that he was okay—I was feeling like I was floating in some other dimension where I had no control over anything. I was agitated and needed someone to hear me—and get my lenses out! Hard gas permeable lenses need to be popped, not pulled out like soft lenses. Somehow, I know I did manage to get them out myself. I still cannot fathom how I did this lying down. I don't recall giving them to the nurse to have them saved for me. I don't know where they got the case to put the lenses in. It was just done. For all I know, angels came down from the heavens and took my lenses out for me.

Once my contacts were out, I could no longer see the clock above the nurse's station clearly. I found something reassuring about that large round clock and the way the second hand moved around the face. It never glided smoothly, but moved forward with a little jerk backwards before proceeding to the next minute line. The clock ticking away assured me that I was still of this world. Clocks were there all through public school, then high school, into college, and in the delivery room when I was in labor, ticking away through key milestones of my life.

The nurse returned with the swabs and asked me to give her my name, date of birth, and age. When I told her I was seventy, she said, "No, my dear, you cannot be seventy years old! All the nurses have been observing you since you were brought down, and even through the bandages on your face, we don't believe you are seventy." Then, as if to be sure, she again asked for my date of birth and how old I was. I refused to answer, reminding her that I had been asked these questions repeatedly. I did not want to answer any more questions!

"What time is it?" I asked.

"About 1:00 a.m. Your surgery is scheduled in about an hour."

"What day is it? What's the date?"

"April 25th, dear."

Too tired to feel much of anything, I was just waiting. I focused my eyes on the clock and, even without my lenses, was able to make out the moving minute hand. It moved ever so slowly. Like my brain. My brain was overloaded, and I could not concentrate. I suppose I should have been fearful or anxious, but I was neither. I only knew I was thankful that I was no longer in horrific pain, was no longer cold, and that the time on the clock was still moving.

CHAPTER 5

THE MORNING
OF APRIL 25TH

I have no recollection of anything else until I woke up in a regular hospital room. In front of me, I was reassured to see the ever-present large clock, with hands on ten and twelve.

I could hear some muffled voices behind a curtain. Then, my beloved's blue eyes appeared, encircled by black-and-blue bruises, with scratched and cut skin above his graying beard. Keith's smile spread comfort through me like a cup of chamomile tea.

"Welcome back, darling. How are you feeling?" he asked as he reached for my hand. His right arm was in a sling, and there was a monitor taped to his chest.

I responded, "Not too sure, but better. How are you?"

"I'm fine."

"Really?" I questioned. "How can you say that? Look at you!" I said, pointing to the monitor on his chest first, and then the sling. "What the fuck happened to us?"

My mind tried to organize and sort out the story. I went to the dentist and fell asleep in the car on the way home. I had an auditory memory of metal scratching, and a video played in my head of the car rotating off the ground. What scared me most at the time was recognizing the absence of Keith.

As I was about to ask Keith questions, Dr. Batman entered the room with several other doctors. "How are you feeling, Elaine?"

As if the question cued me, I wondered: how was I indeed? In the next instant my brain took in a complete body scan, and I was sickened. My legs were slightly elevated, and a sheet covered me from mid-thigh upwards. My left ankle was in a cast that ran partly up my shin, and a large bandage encased my left knee. The cast covered my foot except for the toes, which were a bizarre shade of blue. And I could not wiggle them.

My right leg was held rigid by a metal brace that went from my toes almost to the top of my thigh. There were long thin needles resembling metal skewers inserted into a pink dressing that covered my entire leg. In truth, my leg looked like an animal set for roasting.

My left arm was encircled with a blood pressure cuff that periodically tightened and then loosened as the machine ticked away the numbers. A pole held a tube attached to a bag that deposited fluids slowly dripping into my arm.

My right hand was able to move and, when I raised my arm to check it out, I saw the pinky and ring finger were taped together.

The older of the two other doctors introduced himself as Dr. Miller, an orthopedic surgeon. He was to be operating on me later that afternoon. He introduced his young assistant as Dr. Rosstein. Dr. Miller then looked at Keith.

"I presume this is your husband?" Dr. Miller continued without a pause, "I have a very busy schedule today, so please permit me to speak and then you can ask me any questions." There was no emotion, no kindness in the doctor's script-like recitation. I did not feel much confidence at that point.

"Your legs have the majority of the injuries to your body as a result of the trauma suffered. Your left leg is the better of the two. You have a badly broken ankle, and although the break is bad, it is clean. This means the break itself is like a china plate that has broken in half; it has no splinters. Your leg will eventually repair itself. The cast is to keep it immobile." I tried to interject but he silenced me by putting up his stop-sign hand. "I need to continue. You have had a bad cut to your left knee, and we needed to place twenty-four staples into that area. It will heal nicely.

"The major problem, and the reason for a second surgery, is your right leg. The femur, which is the bone above your knee, has been shattered. This is the strongest bone in your body, and usually there would be a clean break there, but unfortunately, in your case, the bone has shattered. So, I will be putting in a metal plate and screws where there is still bone, to hold the plate in place and keep the bone taut. When I operate, I will also insert pellets of antibiotics with the hope that they will eliminate any bacteria that may cause an infection.

"The bath you had in the ER was an iodine bath, which hopefully took care of the bacteria and, as per the x-rays, washed away all or most of the bone fragments, but we cannot be certain. Not until we can actually examine the bone itself."

Now, Keith interrupted. "What are those metal needles that look like skewers in her leg? What else is wrong with her?"

Dr. Miller looked at Keith, obviously annoyed, but responded, "The skewers, as you call them, will be coming out in surgery. No need to explain what they're for. The other injuries you ask about, well… due to the extreme compression between the seat belt and the airbag, there is severe bruising on her breasts and chest.

"Of course, you can see the lacerations on her face, which were caused by the shattered glass. We have removed all the glass, and the cuts are not deep enough to require stitches. They will need to be kept moist, and we will have a plastic surgeon take a look in a few days. We will also bring in a breast surgeon. Two of her fingers on her right hand have hairline fractures. That is why they are taped together. In a few words? Your wife is lucky to be alive. I have seen the pictures of the accident site."

Dr. Miller moved closer to my bed. "I will now examine her legs. The cast appears too tight. I noticed this earlier. A man called George will be coming in to remove it and reset the cast, so it is not so tight." Turning to me, he said, "Elaine, you'll be getting antibiotics intravenously, along with pain medicine. Unfortunately, you still can't have anything to eat or drink until after the surgery."

Another man entered the room. "This is George," Dr. Miller informed us. "I need to see a few more patients. Unless you have critical questions to ask me, I suggest that we wait to speak again until after the surgery, when there will be more time." And without waiting for a response, he turned and left with his intern.

The last thing I remember from that time was telling George that the new cast still felt too tight. George said he would put some cuts in the new cast, which would help with the pressure.

I seriously have no recollection of anything after that for about a week's time. Nothing at all. Not any of the visitors I was told came to see me. Not Keith in attendance. None of the doctors or nurses.

I remember nothing until May 1st, the evening when our Long Beach friends Shelly and Delores came to visit.

When Keith and I first moved to Long Beach, we met Shelly and Delores at a meeting in the Reform temple. They were somewhat older than us, and we hit it off immediately. Delores was quiet. Shelly, her husband, was a lawyer whose stock-in-trade was his mouth. It was hard for her to get many words in! When we were alone, she was a great conversationalist.

Whenever I looked at Delores, I tried to imagine what she had looked like when she was younger. She was still very striking, with dark hair, almost pure white skin, riveting blue eyes, her face without hardly a wrinkle.

Delores' 1950s-style bangs couldn't hide the look of concern I saw in her eyes when she entered the room. Always stylish, she was dressed to head out to dinner. Normally Keith and I would most likely have been at that table with them. She and Shelly were shocked by what had happened and wanted to do what they could to help.

Shelly, a handsome man with a full head of graying hair, had worked with the American Medical Association during his legal career. He knew all the doctors and hospitals on Long Island, and had put me on some kind of VIP list. Little did we know, his connections and intimate knowledge of the healthcare and insurance systems would prove to be greatly advantageous.

CHAPTER 6

THE BLACK HOLE:
APRIL 26 TO MAY 2

It was the first week of May, and I had come consciously back into my mind after a week of what I call my "dark time". Keith stayed with me through dinner and the shift change of the nurses. He left around 7:30 p.m. after he hugged me and kissed me goodnight. He said he would call me once he got home. It wasn't that he felt he had to report in, but I think he felt that if I knew he was safe, I wouldn't have anything else to worry about except my own healing.

Angela, the night nurse, arrived, checked my blood pressure, gave me my meds, and helped me to roll onto my side so as to put the bedpan underneath me. She warned me, "Keep drinking. You need to keep the fluids up at a maximum to help flush your kidneys. Very important to do this. When the water pitcher is empty, be sure to ring for someone to fill it. I need something from down the hall. Be back in a few to get the pan."

I remembered nothing about ever using a bedpan before, and here Angela was quite comfortable just slipping one under me and walking away. I wondered if I had been using one of these or if there had been a catheter in me during that dark time?

There are all kinds of indignities when you are trapped in a hospital bed. One is being at the mercy of the staff, who walk in and out at all times of the day and night. Nurses, doctors, checking your status; attendants that bring your trays of food and then return to collect them; the cleaners that mop the floors, empty the trash, and clean the bathrooms. Each person has their own job. You could be doing your business on the bedpan and that wouldn't stop anyone from doing what they needed to do to stick to their schedules. There are private rooms at a hospital, but there is no privacy.

The only real benefit I found of private rooms is that you can turn the volume up on the television in order to drown out the other hospital sounds. I found the television instrumental in forcing my brain to shut my body down, so sleep could come. The clock also helped with that, as I could convince my brain it was either midnight or noon, depending upon my preference.

The most ignominy comes from the hospital gown that never seems to fit properly. How could it really? You are trapped in bed, and the only way to get the gown on and off is to be rolled onto one side and then the other. I was glad I only needed to deal with the gown once a day, usually when it (and/or I) needed to be washed and changed.

A stranger, not known to me before but now intimately familiar with all of me, appeared with a pan and warm water, a washcloth, soap, towels, and a new gown. She (usually a she) carried the bedpan with her to be sure the freshly washed sheets and pillowcases would be protected. My regular angel was a slight, young lady named Addie, who couldn't have weighed more than ninety pounds.

Before lowering the bed, Addie would untie the back strings of my gown so I could get my arm out of the sleeve opening. This left me half naked. The bed would then be lowered so that I was nearly flat, and the metal side rail was repositioned. I grabbed the opposite rail with both arms and pulled so that the strength of my one good arm would enable me to get onto my side. My right leg was part of this roll. Addie would wash and dry my back and butt. The same procedure was repeated on the opposite side, but she had to make sure my left leg would not get entangled with my right leg. At this point I would be completely naked. She finished the upper body and left thigh, washed and dried, and then handed me the cloth to do my private parts. A towel covered me while I was manipulated so the sheets and bed pad could be changed. Addie was an expert at pulling and pushing me so a clean gown could ultimately be put on my body until we repeated this routine the next day.

Like the first initial shock of seeing my lower body, the first time I saw my chest I gasped at how black (more than blue), it was from my collar bone to my midsection. I now understood why it hurt so much. The daily rolling from side to side added to the pain. Over time, this subsided into mere discomfort.

Then there was the bedpan routine. I learned not to wait until the last minute to call for the pan, so I could avoid wetting the bed. If I wet the bed, the linens and my gown would need to be changed. Avoiding pain and extra movements became my primary focus. I would make note of the time I called for a pan and see how long it took for someone to respond. And then, once I had completed the task, how long would it take for the pan to be removed? And then I calculated how long, under regular circumstances, I could hold my water. I determined that I needed to use the bedpan at least every two hours. I felt like I was a student doing science experiments and writing a report for school. But at least it was something to focus on besides the television and the gossip of the nurses and staff in the hallway beyond my door.

The urine collection was actually the easy part. The hard part was solid waste. Not only the degradation of using the bedpan once the Colace had done its job, but then to wait until the pan was removed.

All of these manipulations, plus the extent of my bruises and injuries, and the use of bedpans meant there was no way I could wear underwear to cover my bottom. Thus, every time the doctors came to examine me, interns in tow, there was nary a private part of me that wasn't exposed until I could put the gown between my legs. I never lost the feelings of embarrassment.

I remembered when my mother told me to always wear clean underwear, in case I was in an accident. Well, guess what? No one will ever see the underwear, so no need to worry about it! Ha ha ha.

Once I discovered how easy it was for that gown to shift, I got Keith to bring me the sweatshirt I had bought when we went cruising up the Connecticut River. It was soft, longer than standard sweatshirts, very baggy on me, and had buttons so I could close it from the top and bottom as needed. It helped me to control the exposure of my bottom, and the added benefit was that it kept me warm. No number of blankets seemed able to handle that job.

Angela returned. She had forgotten the syringe that held the Heparin needed to stop clots that could form from lack of exercise. She jabbed the needle into my belly and left.

The phone rang, and Keith reassured me, "I'm home, darling. Shelly left a message for me to call tomorrow, early. Maybe he spoke to someone at that AMA dinner and they can admit you to the rehab center? Goodnight. God bless."

"Night, Keith. Take care of yourself. Eat something and rest," I lectured, slipping into my caring wife role. Always worried about the man I love.

I rang for Nurse Angela to come, in the hope she would administer my pain medication early. It had been a miserable day with worsening discomfort from legs to chest, and now my head hurt too. The headache wasn't from the toils of the day but from the journey back to the real world and facing the stark reality that the road back home would take every bit of courage and perseverance I could muster. The pain attached to the injuries would be fixed by drugs. I was not sure how I would cope with the physical trials of getting back up on my feet and, I couldn't help wondering, would being on my feet be the end result or something else?

Looking back, I would have to say that the clock in front of me played a major part in my recovery. I remember late at night, watching the minute hand continuing past the low numbers, then past the higher ones until the minute hand and the hour hand were on top of one another. And once I could see the minute hand had crept past the twelve, I would think to myself, *Here is a clean slate for another day.* Never did I let myself think of the day that had passed, only that there was opportunity for better in the new day.

CHAPTER 7

GRADUATION DAY IN MAY

It was about 6:30 a.m. when Angela peeked in. "Are you awake?" she asked.

"Well, if I wasn't, I am now." I smiled. "I think the nurse who comes to take the blood pressure and my temperature came around five, and I've been up since then. I'm dying for a cup of coffee."

"Breakfast will be up soon. And you, my dear, have a very busy day. Today is your graduation!"

"Graduation?" I mumbled.

"Yup!" she answered, way too enthusiastically for pre-coffee chatter! "We've received orders. First and foremost, I am here to remove the tubes from your arm. You will need to keep the shunt for a while, but all of your meds, including your pain medication, will now be given orally. That should make you feel a lot better. And now that you've become a pro, you will be giving yourself the needles in your belly. You've successfully passed that course with flying colors!"

"You will need to prepare all of your personal things because you will be moving down to the rehab floor in the afternoon. Before then you are going to have pictures taken."

"Pictures? Graduation?" I questioned. I was so confused.

"Well, it's not what you think," she smiled. "These pictures will be taken by the radiologist who will send them to your doctor—who, by the way, is expected to see you after the x-rays. He will be here to remove the staples from your left knee. I see by the chart that there are twenty-four staples, so best that you count them to be sure he didn't miss any. Only joking," she assured me quickly when she saw the dismay creeping into my face. "And of course, he's going to check the cast again."

"What about the pain in my rear end?" I whined.

"You have had no activity for many days. Without activity, the muscles lose their strength and size, and the bones become more prominent, but that will all change once you are in rehab."

"And what about my right leg?" I asked.

"No notations on the chart about that, deary. Best you speak to the doctor when he gets here."

At this point, her tone and face became more serious, and she took my hand. "I've been taking care of patients in this trauma hospital for many years. Here's my advice. Rehab will not be easy. Do not push yourself in the beginning. Rehab is a slow process. Do not, I repeat, DO NOT overdo. And do not be discouraged. Think of your body as a jigsaw puzzle, with a thousand pieces. In the beginning, it's hard to find the corners. Once you have them, you can do many things. Work towards getting the pieces on the edges, even put together some pieces in the middle because you're learning how to look for the pieces you need. Eventually the pieces will start to form a recognizable picture. And it is not uncommon to feel frustrated because things don't line up as you expect them to. But you know, with patience and time, the picture will be completed."

Changing her tone and smiling, Angela continued, "You must have high connections here because you will have your own room down on the rehab floor.

"You might want to call your husband and let him know where to find you. If he comes up here and finds the bed empty and your stuff gone, we don't want him to panic!" she said, half joking. "Remember, he's recovering too!"

And so, the next phase began. Once the tubes were removed from my arms, an orderly pushed the bed to the elevator. The orderly guided me out of the elevator, past a desk where several nurses were doing paperwork, to a station where they signed me in. I was repositioned outside the x-ray room to wait my turn.

Once I was inside, the technician smiled, bowed a little, introduced himself, and welcomed me. He and my erstwhile chauffeur grabbed the edges of the sheets and lifted me off the bed and onto the x-ray table. It was like being in a hammock, but the hammock was not the gentle swaying kind at a beachfront resort, but more like a hammock caught in a hurricane. It was by no means gentle, and I kept imagining myself being dropped. I guess, under the circumstances, it was at least effective.

The surface of the x-ray table upon which I was deposited was freezing cold and as hard as a slab of marble. I could feel the bones in my rear end rebelling. Is it horrible to say that at that moment I was envious of my friends with more ample bottoms? My right heel (the only part of my leg not covered by the brace) connected with the cold metal, sending tiny electric shocks down into my toes.

I began to hyperventilate. I felt I was on the precipice of an asthma attack, but it never quite developed.

The breakfast tray was waiting for me when I got back to my room, but after the "swinging" time I had just experienced, I had lost my appetite.

It was orthopedic surgeon, Dr. Martin and his assistant who came visiting about an hour after the x-rays were taken. Just taking the x-rays had been very scary. I had no recollection of x-rays being taken before, and thus I didn't know what to expect when they were compared.

"I've seen the x-rays and your ankle is healing nicely. The cast will need to remain for several more weeks, at least until we see that the bones are 80 percent healed. Then it can come off. The physical therapy will help you regain some of the strength in your upper leg. This will be of enormous help once you are standing and then walking. When the cast comes off, you will be in a brace for support, but in my opinion, from what I see, it won't take too long before that leg and your ankle are back to normal."

"What about my right leg?"

"I am now going to change the dressing."

"But," I pushed, "what did you see when you looked at that x-ray?"

His look was one of concern. "The injuries sustained were extensive. The femur is the largest bone in the body and the strongest. In your case, the femur shattered. The second operation I performed was to align the bone. I had to try to find enough bone, and then anchor in a metal plate and screws. There are eight screws. The best way I can describe your bone to you is to think of a piece of aged Swiss cheese. At present, it is difficult to make any appraisal of your right leg's condition, even comparing it to the other pictures we have.

"There will be very limited physical therapy on that right leg, except for this. Every day, twice a day, you will go on a machine that will bend your right knee. Each session will be two hours. This is needed to break up the scar tissue. That knee needs to work properly in order to be able to walk properly. In the beginning, you will also need to strengthen your arms and back muscles while working on your left leg. You will need the strength to get from the bed to the wheelchair, and to get onto the beds and chairs in the rehab room. The head of the physical therapy department will be in to see you once you are moved downstairs. You will like her. All my patients do."

The doctor told me I would continue to wear the brace on my right leg. The brace went from the ankle all the way to my upper thigh. There was a clamp with a dial at the knee, so there was a small amount of movement. When I was in bed, the leg was somewhat straight in front of me. When I was in a wheelchair, the chair arms were down, the footrest on the left side was out so my left leg could rest on it, and my right leg was extended, almost like it was in bed, so it wouldn't touch the floor.

I could not bear to watch as Dr. Miller re-dressed my leg. I did not want to see it, not at that time, so I closed my eyes.

There was just too much to think about, much too much to digest. For the first time, I thought about the possibility of never being able to get out of the bed. Or perhaps being in a wheelchair for the rest of my life. Being a cripple. (God, I hate that word.) *Think of something pretty*, I told myself. And I did. I conjured up the same scene I used during my divorce when I needed to relax and get through rough times.

I'm at a picnic with a few good friends, laughing and happy. We're sitting alongside a wonderful, slow-flowing river. The trees are blooming; vibrant flowers surround us.

I breathed into this image and was able to open my eyes. Dr. Miller was done and said he would visit me in a few days. The assistant would be stopping by to see me every day.

As Dr. Miller turned to leave, I mustered all my courage and called out, "Wait, before you go. Will I eventually be able to walk again?"

"Take one day at a time, Elaine. We need to see how well you do with the physical therapy, what needs to be done for any possible infection, and how quickly some of the more minor injuries that you sustained heal." Pausing, and taking a deep breath, he looked into my eyes and said, "It is my hope that the answer will be yes. Remember what I told you. The injury to your right leg is extensive. Stay positive!"

The clock said it was only 10:30 a.m. It seemed as if a lot more time had passed since Angela had walked in earlier that morning.

The day nurse came into my room and introduced herself. Suzanne advised me that I had about an hour before I would be moving to the rehab floor. One of the orderlies would be coming to pack up my stuff, and take me and the bed downstairs.

Rehab was on the 8th floor. *That's good*, I thought. When my career in international freight business took me to China, my contacts had told me years ago that eight was a lucky number. Maybe because it looked like infinity? The thought of being on the lucky floor lifted my spirits a bit.

My new room was at the end of the hallway, past the elevator. It was smaller than my previous room and had only one bed. I was relieved, as I didn't think I could stand having a roommate. I had enough to cope with on my own.

The window looked out on the main street. Something to distract me besides the television and clock.

The transfer from my old bed to the new bed went without a hitch. And just as I was settling in, the old bed being pushed out of the room, in walked two women dressed in green scrubs. One was pushing a wheelchair and I thought, *Here we go!*

CHAPTER 8

REHAB BEGINS

9 DAYS SINCE THE ACCIDENT

"Hello there. Welcome to rehab. I'm Carol, the rehab supervisor, and this is Iona, the therapist assigned to your case. You will be seeing a lot of us from now on. We'll be working as a pair in the beginning and, as you can see, we have brought you your chariot," she said showing off my shiny new wheelchair with a sweeping motion like Vanna White on *Wheel of Fortune*. The "chariot" was laden with a six-inch thick cushion and on top of the seat was a wooden board. This board was very narrow and shiny, about three and a half feet long, and my thoughts went from wondering if we would be playing wheelchair cricket to if this was some kind of corporal punishment device.

Carol was about 5'5" with dark brown hair, and fairly big boned. She had a welcoming smile and twinkling blue eyes. I liked her immediately. I estimated her age around forty-five to fifty years.

Iona was taller, perhaps 5'8", blonde hair, blue eyes, very thin, and somewhere in the neighborhood of thirty years old.

Carol shared that Iona was from Sweden and had been with the hospital for a year or so. Iona had come to the USA to do specialized training, so she could get certified when she returned to Sweden. "She is an excellent therapist, and all of our patients just love her," Carol enthused. "Well," she added with a wink, "patients love me too!"

"You will have occupational therapy once daily and physical therapy once daily. You are probably familiar with physical therapy but perhaps not occupational therapy?" Carol continued, "As you have been virtually inactive for about ten days, you are in a situation where most of your muscles have deteriorated from lack of use. So many things that were natural for you to do prior to your accident, you no longer have the strength to do. We'll guide you through a series of exercises to strengthen your upper body, especially your arms. Your arms will be the vehicle to get you in and out of bed and into the wheelchair, as well as from the wheelchair to the bed or chairs in rehab, and of course onto and off the toilet. Later on, we'll work with you on how to put your brace on and take it off.

"The good news is that now that you're on the rehab floor, you can feel like your life is starting to become more normal again. You'll be able to enjoy some of our classes and play games with your visitors or other patients. We offer painting, sewing, crafts, and games like Scrabble, Monopoly, or cards. Part of occupational therapy is to discuss your fears and how to overcome them. You will be meeting with several of our other staff, who will assist you with both physical and occupational therapy.

"Regarding physical therapy, your first session will be tomorrow morning," Carol kept going. "This afternoon, Iona and I will be

here to show you how to use this board, and you'll get your first lesson in moving on it. You'll be able to get from bed to the wheelchair
and back again. In a very short time, you will be able to do this on
your own with no supervision. You'll also do exercises today in the
occupational therapy room that are designed to improve your upper
body strength. Not to worry; you won't ever look like a weight-
lifter," she concluded, half smiling.

The verbal instruction manual continued with notification that
Iona would be taking me to therapy rooms in the morning and
afternoon, and would assist me in practicing to get on and off the
board, into and out of bed and wheelchair. I was told that a very
strong female attendant would be helping me with toileting, which
meant I would finally be rid of the bedpan, except for overnight.

Once the informational and introductory portion of the lecture
was over, Carol said we would be starting on my first two-hour session, in which we'd be working to break up scar tissue in my knee.

"You will be able to bend your knee much more than you are able
to do now. Eventually you need to get your knee to a ninety-degree
angle. Okay," She smiled as she pulled back the sheet and placed
my braced right leg onto the board. "—let's see what your right knee
can do. Go as far as you can by sliding your foot on this board, moving your heel towards your backside. When you stop, I will measure
the angle. Then, using all your will power and strength, let's see if
you are in pain, and how much more you can do!"

Try as I could, the knee hardly bent at all. Not so good.

Carol, no longer businesslike, took my hand and kindly said,
"The staff on this floor are very different from the hospital floor. We
understand about trauma and the trials ahead of you, the difficulties
you will encounter. Our job is to get you out of this hospital as soon
as possible by building your strength and your confidence, so that

once you are at home, you will be able to function within certain parameters. We'll be back later. Enjoy your lunch."

A new chapter was now beginning, and I focused on telling myself not to be afraid. I almost laughed aloud when the thought crossed my mind, an old gym saying, "no pain, no gain." I sort of knew that the pain would probably increase, but I don't think I was really prepared for it. In fact, I was definitely not prepared for it!

I had already called Keith on my cell phone to let him know about being moved to the rehab floor. With my personal property finally secured in my new room, I advised Keith of where I was and the schedule ahead of me for the afternoon. He wished me good luck and said he was bringing dinner and a visitor. My son David was on a flight from Miami to JFK! He was to be up in New York for a few days and would be there for my first actual physical therapy session. My son David is a gym nut and has worked with several different trainers. I thought it would be excellent to have his input about the overall plan they devised for me. I hadn't seen David in several months and had only spoken to him a few times since the accident.

Carol and Iona returned around 1:00 p.m. They handed me back the board.

"This is your new best friend, and your second new best friend is that wheelchair," Carol said. "You need to sit up nice and straight and pay attention. The first thing you will need to do is use the remote to reposition the bed so it is only slightly higher than the chair. I am going to do that for you now, so that you can see where the cushion is, relative to the bed. You will then place the board like so." She demonstrated how to position the board as a bridge from the bed to the cushion on the chair. "You have to remember to lock the brake first."

"And then what?" I asked.

"And then you will need to use your arms to get your butt onto the board, and be able to use your arms to slide along the board onto the cushion."

"Uhm. You've got to be joking!" I said, looking from the bed to the board to the chair skeptically.

Carol ignored my remark. (*How many times had she heard that before!?*)

"The chair," she continued, "is positioned so that your right leg will be the one that is transferred first, giving you the ability to control movement with your left leg and your arms." My right leg was in the brace and was able to bend slightly. It wasn't extended in front of me as I feared. Carol then paused, looked at me seriously (like a schoolteacher lecturing an errant child), and said, "You can NEVER, and I repeat, NEVER, allow your right leg to have any weight on it, at all! The doctor has told us that if there is even the *slightest* bit of weight on your right leg, there is a distinct possibility that the bone will further shatter and, if that happens, you might not ever be able to walk again."

It was as if the last few words were in all capital letters.

NEVER BE ABLE TO WALK AGAIN.

I started to sweat profusely and felt sick to my stomach. My breath came in short bursts as I looked around for a pail. Iona shouted to put my head down, and she put an ice pack on my neck. Carol gave me some ice water, instructing me to take small sips.

"You know this is not going to be easy," Carol said, in a kinder tone. "You need to trust us, and trust in yourself that you have the ability to do what is necessary to get well and get you out of here. Now, take some deep breaths and count slowly to ten. Put your hands on the board and get familiar with how it feels. The chair is positioned correctly, it's locked, and we are going to hold you. I promise, you will not fall. Your arms are strong enough to get you moving along the board, and we'll be helping you."

To me, the short space between the mattress edge and the cushion may well have been the distance between the sides of the Grand Canyon. I was scared to death! I had been in a bed, except for the trip for x-rays, forever, it felt like. One part of me was pushing me to stay where I was, while another part of me was pushing me to go forward, or in this case, sideways.

With my heart pounding in my ears and sweat filling my armpits, I pushed myself so that my body was angled at the side of the mattress, and I managed to get my butt on the board. Iona was in front of me and had hold of my legs. Carol was somewhere behind me, with a tight grip on my right arm and shoulder. "Now, get your right arm moving along that board. Your body will follow."

I was half on the bed, half on the seat of the wheelchair, and then a miracle happened... I was in the wheelchair! Carol smiled broadly.

"Well done!" She enthused.

"Lift your butt so I can remove the board. Use your arms to center yourself on the seat," she instructed.

Iona placed my right leg gently onto the footrest while I was able to get my left foot onto the footrest by myself. Carol demonstrated how to get the wheelchair arm down and undo the brake. Carol said, "How do you feel?"

I answered, a little shaky but smiling, "I am not sure."

"You should feel proud of yourself! For a first try, aside from the panic, you did well! Really well!"

CHAPTER 9

Occupational Therapy

Iona wheeled me down to the room where I was to have my first occupational therapy session. The first exercises were for arm strengthening. I used an arm bike, rotating clockwise and then counterclockwise to complete the number of rotations assigned. Not too bad. I was a little sore.

Then, onto a weight machine. This was to assist in strengthening my upper arms and shoulders. Again, not too bad.

When I completed these two exercises, Carol came over and said, "I am taking you over to the table and we are going to see how you do to stand up." When she said this, I felt a little faint. Especially after having been given the warning about not putting any weight at all on my right foot.

She and Iona placed the wheelchair so my knees were just at the edge of the table, pushed the footrests out, which allowed my feet to dangle not too far off the floor. The pair stood on either side of me.

"Use your arms to push yourself forward until I tell you to stop," Carol said. "Bend your left knee, so your foot is flat on the floor. The brace on your right leg will not allow your foot to drop. Hold on to the table edge now, with both hands. Iona and I will hold onto your arms and shoulders. Do not let go. Now, up you go!"

And there I was, standing on one leg, looking like the Karate Kid about to do a crane kick. My whole body was trembling. Primarily I think it was fear, more than my muscles rebelling, that made me tremble.

I spent ten seconds (according to my beloved clock) on my one foot, and then they lowered me down. Iona gave me some cold water. She told me I did fine and promised that in a few days I would able to do this by myself. My first instinct was to feel skeptical, but then I realized that each thing they told me I'd be able to do, I did. So why not be confident in myself? I resolved to focus and put my best effort forward.

"Carol and I (or maybe another therapist) will have a grip on you, but we won't be using our strength to get you up. Now, we are going to repeat the same thing we just did. Are you ready?"

And up I went. It was easier this time, as there was less fear. The third time up was quicker. I imagined my muscles were speaking to one another saying, *I remember how we do this.*

When I returned to my room, Carol and Iona left me in the wheelchair and said I needed to get used to sitting up. They left the brake off and Carol suggested, "Experiment a bit with the chair, see how to go forwards and backwards and how to turn around. We'll be back in about half an hour, and then you'll learn how to use the slide board to get back to bed. It will be more difficult than getting out, as gravity will not be helping you."

I called Keith to let him know I was back in my room and that the first session went okay. Then I told him how hard it was getting up on my one foot and how much my body had rebelled.

"I am so proud of you, babe," he said. "We will conquer this. I love you. See you later."

He told me Shelly and Dolores would be coming the next night to look in on me, and that he would call me before he left the office. He then let me know that David's plane was on time.

In the whole of our time together, when faced with any kind of adversity, Keith and I always faced it as "we." We were like Tweedle Dee and Tweedle Dum; two independent bodies .always thinking and acting like one. That was us now, but it didn't start out that way.

CHAPTER 10

KEITH & ELAINE, THE BEGINNINGS

In the beginning of our relationship, Keith used to refer to me as his wounded bird. My divorce had left me quite vulnerable, but I don't think I knew just how vulnerable I really was. I used to kid him that he managed to take a wounded bird and turn her into an eagle.

Well, at that moment in the hospital, I didn't feel like an eagle. I was back to feeling like that wounded bird, especially emotionally. *Okay*, I said to myself. *David will be coming.* My sons had never seen me as anything but strong and confident, and giving up was not in my nature.

In the summer of 1980, I was dating a man who invited me to spend the weekend with him in Montauk, a beach town at the end of Long Island, New York. He told me I would be on my own Saturday night because he would be meeting some of his buddies for night fishing. "You can drop me at 7:00, pick me up 1:00 a.m. and except for those few hours, I'll show you the best time ever."

I agreed.

Two boats went out. Only one was at dockside at 1:00 a.m, and fifteen minutes later, still no second boat. I was getting concerned, so I went into the bar to see what I could find out. A man sitting at the bar told me he was waiting for his brother and that boat was always late, as it went a bit farther out. "How about I buy you a drink?"

"Fine," I said.

He told me he was a clairvoyant and proceeded to tell me all about my auras and what the colors meant. He then told me my mother, who lived in Florida, was doing fine. I had said nothing to him about anything, so how could he know that?

The last thing he said was that I wouldn't be dating the man I was waiting for much longer. "You will spend the next six months not dating at all. And then you will meet a man—blond hair, blue eyes, thirty-four years old, from across the sea, with a beard—and you will be with him for the rest of your life."

At that moment we heard the soft toot of the arriving boat. He handed me his card, saying, "Tell all your friends about me."

And it all happened just the way he told me.

It was Thursday, March 12, 1981, when my friend Paul called to invite me for dinner to meet his friend and colleague, who had recently arrived from the UK.

"I can't," I said. "I fell down two flights of stairs this morning at the Long Island Railroad Station. I look like something out of a horror show, and I am in a lot of pain."

"How'd that happen?"

"My heel got stuck in a crack. I started to fall forward, and when I reached for the bannister to break my fall, it flipped me over onto my face. I am all banged up, scrapes all over. What saved me, I think, was my winter coat. Anyway, my shoe is still in the crack, waiting for Prince Charming to find it and me."

"Sorry," Paul said. "Let me know if there's anything you need. But, you do have to meet my friend. He's very depressed. And you're the best antidepressant I know. He's threatening to cancel his contract and go back to the UK."

"No," I repeated.

But Paul didn't give up. He called three more times that night, begging me to see his friend.

Finally, I said, "Okay. Okay. But let him know I don't even look human. And I have nothing in the house to drink, so if he wants something more than coffee, he'll have to bring it. Tell him to come tomorrow night, around eight, and he can stay one hour, no more."

I could actually hear Paul smile as he hung up the phone.

When I woke in the morning, my face had started to turn a shade of blue around all the red bruises. My lips were swollen as was my face. The scrapes really didn't look good at all. With my white winter skin, the red-and-blue bruises, I looked like some distorted version of an American flag. And I was supposed to meet someone?

My young boys must have heard me moaning as I looked into the mirror because they knocked on the bathroom door.

"Hey, Ma. Are you okay? Open up and let's see what you look like."

When I opened the door, they both looked confused and seemed to be alternating between laughing or crying. Both of them told me they would not stay after school but would come directly home.

It was my son David, the younger of the two, who reminded me that it was Friday the 13th as he ran for his camera to get my face on film. Why? So, he could make up his face on Halloween to look exactly like I did! And could I get him a cast for his arm, he wanted to know. It was painful but I started laughing, and tears ran out of my eyes. Boys!

My friend Joe was an orthopedic surgeon. He called in a prescription for pain medication after hearing the tale of my "down-fall." He advised me that if I could move everything on my body, there was probably nothing broken but that I should call and check in with him the following morning.

After the boys left for school, I got into a warm bath, hoping it would help me remove the remainder of the nylon threads from my pantyhose that were embedded into my scrapes. It was slow going.

As the day passed, not only did the pain increase, but so did the swelling. The patriotic colors of my face turned more into the rainbow nation. Joe had told me that the pain would intensify for the first three days and then dissipate. He recommended applying ice on the bruises.

The boys decided to have dinner with their father, and I was alone when the doorbell rang. I had completely forgotten that I had agreed to see Paul's friend, who was standing there, liquor bottle in hand.

Paul's friend was tall, with blond hair and blue eyes. He was clean shaven.

"Hi," I said. "Sorry. I'm not dressed for a visitor. I just didn't have the right outfit to go with my face."

He laughed. "It's not that bad." And I was immediately charmed by his British accent.

"Liar, liar. Come on in."

"Just in case you don't remember, my name is Keith."

"Sit down," I said, pointing to the living room couch. "I'll get you a glass. Do you want ice? I'm on painkillers and antibiotics, not drinking." As I handed him the glass, I added, "Tell me a little about yourself." I let him know that when the pain pill kicked in, I'd be able to participate in the conversation.

Over the next hour, Keith told me about how he and Paul had become friends in the UK. That they had worked for the same company there, that he had taken the position of UK route manager, and was now on a four-year visa to work in the States.

I told him that I was divorced, with two sons, and blurted out my age. I don't know why I told him. Must have been the loosening of lips from the painkillers.

He said he loved older women, and we both laughed. I was thirty-nine to his thirty-four.

Keith checked off all the boxes, except for the beard, of the clairvoyant's description of my life partner. Later, Keith did grow a beard. I eventually told Keith about the prediction and we occasionally referred to it as an anchor of knowing we were meant to be, and that we would get through anything together.

Every year after that first meeting, we celebrated Friday the 13th as our special day.

CHAPTER 11

DAVID VISITS

Keith came in first; he hugged and kissed me. I could see by the look on David's face he was shocked when he saw me. He had never seen me confined to bed.

When David was about four, after I had gotten my older son Mitch out the door for school, I just wasn't feeling well, and I said to myself, *David is still sleeping. Maybe if I lie down for a while, I will feel better.*

Next thing I knew I was being poked, hard! I let out a scream. There was David with a broomstick in his hand.

"I thought you were dead," he sobbed.

"Why would you think that?" I said, wiping his tears and trying to calm him down.

"You're always up. Always, Mama."

"Well," David said, "you don't look all that bad. Will there be any scarring on your face?"

"Don't think so," I replied.

He asked if I could pull back the covers so he could see my legs. I did.

He remarked about the cast and the rough red scar on my left knee. When he looked at the brace, he asked, "Are the stitches out?"

"Not yet, but soon, they tell me."

He told me he had spoken to his trainer, and he had some idea of what would go on in the physical therapy room the next day. He let me know that he wanted to question the therapists as to the overall plan and the exercises. He asked me about the wheelchair and the board.

"The board you see on the wheelchair is so I can use my arms to slide from the bed to the chair and back, and then to other places, like the wheelchair to the toilet.

"They are going to bring in a CPM machine tonight around eight. It's some kind of mechanical device that will move my knee. It's supposed to break up some of the scar tissue. I cannot move my leg at all. Not even from the hip," I said softly. "I can move my toes though. And my ankle, a little bit. But I think that the ankle is more restricted by the brace. I did stand up on my left leg today for a few seconds, and hopefully I will be able to do more.

"I am off the bedpan now, so they tell me. I have yet to be on the toilet, but they tell me the night nurse will treat me to that experience tonight. That should be interesting. At least I know what to do in there. Many, many years of experience." And the three of us laughed.

I explained everything that had happened since the accident, but I found all of the questions (and even just having a conversation) really exhausting. The more I had to repeat all of the gory details, the more I got depressed.

"Mom, Keith and I need to be going soon. I was up early and I'm tired, but I will be here first thing tomorrow morning. I'll bring bagels and cream cheese so you can have a nice breakfast with me. I intend to be here most of the morning, and then I'll go to the office. I'll be back in the evening." He hugged me and whispered in my ear, "You're going to be fine, just fine."

Keith hugged me too, saying they were going to get a bite at the diner, and then home to Long Beach. Keith looked at me with such sadness in his eyes. I couldn't even begin to imagine what he was going through.

The CPM machine arrived around 9:30 p.m., just after one of the nurses had taken me to the toilet. This was to ensure that I could sit with the machine for the full two continuous hours without needing bathroom breaks. The pain medication had been administered at 9:00 p.m. so that its effects would be at full capacity.

CPM stands for Continuous Passive Motion. It was a long metal box, lined with sheepskin, and had several straps placed strategically so that my leg would not shift. The plan was to bend and straighten my knee at prescribed angles. It had a dial, which had a counter from 1–90. It was set at 30 to start. This was the angle between being level and being raised. I needed to increase that angle to 90 degrees so I could go home. The machine would go with me.

The timing of the up and down was automatically set. At 30 degrees, the pain wasn't too bad. As the angle increased, so did the pain. On that first night, it was the nurse who came in to adjust the angle. I was told that in a few days, I would be the one to increase the angle myself. All I could do was watch the television to distract myself, but it didn't help. Maybe once the stitches were out (which was supposed to happen first thing in the morning) it would be better? I hoped. I never did stop hating that medieval torture machine.

Sleep came easier that night. However, nightmares woke me up many times, as did my own tears. I wondered if I would be able to

get through the next day, especially not knowing what would happen in the physical therapy room.

I soothed myself with the thought that David would be there to
help and guide me, to encourage me and keep me from giving into
the fear and the pain. And mostly, to take the burden off Keith.

CHAPTER 12

REHAB, DAY 2

Hospitals are not a place where you can rest. At least not in rehab. When you have a cold or flu the doctor tells you to rest, stay in bed, drink lots of fluids, take Tylenol for a fever, and one duly complies. Lack of sleep was not a problem, because most of the time, due to the painkillers and other drugs, I was out of it anyway. My sleep just wasn't all in one solid block of time.

In between the nightmares that awakened me that first night and the nurse who came in several times to take my vitals, I had maybe three hours of sleep total. My average sleep time before the accident was about five hours. If I ever slept longer than that, I was not functioning as well. This had been the case ever since I was a teenager.

I wondered if the nurses had been trained by army drill sergeants. Never having been in the army, I didn't know how they got you up to start your day. In the old movies, they would blow a bugle, and the drill sergeant marched in, barked out a command, and somehow the soldiers would be lined up, dressed, beds made, and at the ready in a flash.

It was about 5:30 a.m. when I heard the night nurse pushing a machine ever closer to my room, the high-pitched squeak of its wheels sounding like fingernails scratching on a blackboard. When the night nurse came in, she flipped on the piercing fluorescent lights. The machine she brought was meant to test your vitals, to see if you were still alive I suppose, but you would think she'd know I was awake and alive based on my jerky movements trying to block the light, and the moans I shared for all my neighbors to hear. No chance to beg for five more minutes. No snooze alarms. Everyone has a job to do. My job was to suck it up!

As she checked my vitals and made notations in my chart, the nurse offered some helpful (and anxiety provoking) suggestions.

"Your surgeon called, said he had an early surgery and would be here about 8:30 a.m. to take the staples out of your left leg. After the amount of time you've spent here, your leg will in no way resemble the leg you had before the accident. If you have the courage, you can look. If you do decide to look, I suggest you might want to go light on the breakfast; many patients gag or throw up. I go off shift about 7:30, and as my day off is tomorrow, you won't see me tomorrow night."

I asked her if she would send in an attendant who could help me into the bathroom, so I could go potty. It was not easy to manipulate the wheelchair in small spaces, so an attendant was required to put the wheelchair in the optimal position to facilitate my use of the slide board. I supposed this also cut down on the hospital's liability from people falling when trying to get onto the toilet.

Getting me into the bathroom to do my business was easier than getting me out. Once seated on the toilet, I noticed that there was a tiny plastic square on the wall, attached to a plastic string, with a sign that read *pull to call attendant*. Pulling that cord was one thing; getting a response was quite another. The arrival of someone, especially during a shift change, was always a question of patience.

The clock read 6:00 a.m., and I decided to remain in the wheel-chair instead of getting back into the bed. Painful as it was on my buttocks, at least the pain was in a different spot.

That spot reminded me of the times I spent cold winter days sitting on the metal bleachers after school, watching the boys play football, as my bones shivered, trying to escape out of my numb, frozen body.

I don't recollect the exact time I started thinking about how the mind controls the body, but it was definitely before the doctor arrived and before my cell phone pinged with a message from David that he was delayed and would come in the afternoon instead of the morning.

National Geographic magazine had an article quoting scientists, claiming that humans only use about 5 percent of our brain. I calcu-lated that if I could focus my concentration, I could force my brain to send a message to the muscles and ligaments in my dead leg and maybe, just maybe, I could get it to move. My plan was to direct that message to my legs at least fifty times a day. I needed to do that from the wheelchair as it would undoubtedly be harder for my leg to move when it was level to the mattress. I was so intent on taking this action strategy to help heal my wounded body, that when the doctor walked into my room, it didn't even register with me.

When he began to examine me, I didn't look. I didn't even feel anything except a tugging. He said that the scar from the surgery was healing nicely. No sign of any infection, he assured me. He ordered a cream for the nurse to apply, to diminish the size and redness of the scar.

We then discussed my rehab and he said that if all went accord-ing to plan, maybe I could go home in about a week. I was over-joyed! I determined I would do whatever was required to make this happen. He cautioned me that I MUST, and he emphasized again,

I MUST get the angle of my thigh to knee to 90 degrees. And he finished up with a big smile, telling me I could have a shower the next day. (Amazing how the things I would get excited about had changed in just a few weeks!)

My schedule was to spend four hours daily on the CPM machine, not including the time to set it up. I would spend two hours in the morning and two hours in the evening. I would also spend two hours in the rehab room with the therapists and at least one or two hours doing other exercises. There would be enough quiet time to do my brain muscle messaging.

As was now my habit, the morning was spent doing arm exercises. I was doing more reps at the same tension and weight. Carol motioned me to the table, where I would get up on my one good leg.

I'm not entirely sure if practice makes perfect, but I am sure that when the mind can assess the degree of fear and deal with it, the fear itself diminishes. On this, my second full day of physical therapy, I was prepared. I knew what to expect. Carol again advised me that she and Iona would be at my side to assist me to stand up, but this time she asked me to close my eyes, take some really deep breaths, and then to breathe normally. When I was ready, I was to say so.

"Remember," Iona said, "you must grip the table edge tightly, push forward on the chair, and push as hard as you can to get your leg to use its power to straighten itself out, so you can stand on that one leg. Be mindful that the brace is locked at the knee, so there's no chance of your right leg hitting the floor. We will be here to give you the added push, if you need it."

"Ready," I said. And up I went. Painful as it was, the tremors were not as intense and seemed to end more quickly, compared to the previous day. Up we went again. And once more for a third time. "Excellent!" they both cheered in unison.

Carol said, "Iona will walk with you, but we want you to wheel yourself back to your room. Be mindful of the direction and where your room is. When you get tired, let Iona know. And don't push it. At least not today."

I was making progress and improving. It felt good. I was really proud of myself and very encouraged.

Just as we rolled into my room, there was my nurse with my drugs.

The CPM machine was about to arrive, and I was told to get into bed. Iona supervised me on the slide board. I was getting the hang of transferring from surface to surface. (Too much self-congratulations?)

The CPM angle was set on 65. It had been about thirty minutes since I had taken the pain pills. As the machine started to bend my knee, electric shocks rippled through my body. It was as if my body remembered what it had gone through when they gave me the iodine bath in the ER. "Stop it! Stop it!" I shouted to the attendant.

"Listen, young lady," he said sternly. "If you ever want to get up and get out of here, you have to get this to 90 degrees, and 55 won't cut it. I will leave it on 55 and be back in thirty minutes to turn it up."

I kept my eyes on the clock. The turn-it-up phase wasn't too successful. The attendant put it to 60. Sixty was painful, although less so due to the oxycodone or Percocet that kicked in, and I kept myself distracted by watching television. The attendant said, "You have to do this to break up the scar tissue. I am setting it to 65. You have to withstand it for at least five minutes, so bear up."

The second hand was just moving ever so slowly. It seemed at times to be standing still. I even imagined that it was going backwards, just for spite!

My mind spun with thoughts about the hospital pushing me out and I would be a cripple for the rest of my life. *Cripple.* The word made my stomach turn. Five minutes seemed like an eternity. Then the machine relaxed the angle. I breathed in and out. Then he pushed it back again to 65. The pain was excruciating. And then, "Thank God." That was finally over. Two hours of intense torture. I didn't think I could go on. Wasn't the trauma of the accident enough?

My chest still hurt, and the bruises had faded to a charming eggplant purple. My face had red lines wherever the shards of glass had been, like I had been in a fight with a frenzied cat. Maybe the staff lied to me and I would need plastic surgery? The reality of my situation was sinking in, and I thought maybe it would have been better if I hadn't survived. And then I remembered my messaging. I gave myself a little pep talk.

"Okay, Elaine. Give it a try. If it works, well it works. Pray it works."

At the end of the two-hour morning CPM torture session, it was time for lunch. I transferred myself back to the wheelchair. I began my messaging. The first of the fifty I had promised myself to deliver to my body every day. It wasn't like the command in David Bowie's *Space Oddity* at all. No Major Tom here. I just closed my eyes and gently pretended I was speaking to a small baby (not unlike a new mother facing her baby with an outstretched arm holding a toy). "Okay, now, you can do it; let go; walk to me…"

"Okay, brain… sending a message to my right leg to make it move." Nothing. Twenty thoughts later, still nothing. I stopped when David arrived.

"Hi, Mom. Sorry for the delay in getting here," he apologized as he looked me over. "Well, you don't look so bad today."

"Thanks," I said sarcastically. He came over and hugged me very gently.

"I stopped by the desk. Your therapy is in about fifteen minutes. I asked if I could take you there. Let's see how you drive those wheels," he said, smiling. I went down the corridor, propelling forward by using my upper body strength to push the metal hand rim around the tires, making note of how to get to therapy from my room.

As we traversed the hallway, David coached me. "Remember when I had my football accident? Even though the injury to my back didn't allow me to play football any longer, all the physical therapy has allowed me to exist pretty normally. I have pain, but working with a trainer keeps it under control. You need to push, and if it is painful, well then, TOUGH! I want you out of this bed. I want you up and running around with your grandchildren. Look at what you've accomplished in your life already! I have always seen you determined to succeed. No matter what you had to do, or the price, and this is no different. I know you can do it!"

We met one of the therapists, Charlie, on the way in. She didn't look like a Charlie to me. She was very slight. She directed me to a line of chairs and said she would be back shortly.

David and I looked around the room. It was a large space, brightly lit with afternoon sun. I noticed eight green, leather covered, padded beds (aka tables), all of which had seen better days. One wall had a rack of rubber balls of assorted sizes and colors. Hooks held various colors of hanging rubber bands. And while this looked like the grown-up version of a kindergarten play area, I would eventually make use of all of these tools and learn that playing with these "toys" was going to improve my strength. Plenty of water stations were set up around the room, and everyone seemed to have a water bottle handy. Hydration, I learned, is as important to bone and muscle recovery as it is to keeping your digestive system functioning well.

My eyes focused on an elderly woman being assisted by two therapists who wanted her to try walking between two parallel bars. She kept slipping and crying, losing her balance, even though the therapist were holding her to keep her upright. I vowed that wasn't going to be me!

There were other people around with braces like mine and plenty of people with casts sitting in a row, waiting their turn. Some people were doing a variety of exercises, and others were just sitting and staring into space.

David took this time for more pep talk. "Look around. There are many here in worse condition than you are. Think about how lucky you are to still be alive, and have your brain still working, and no facial scarring. You need to promise me that you'll do everything to get back to your old self, physically and mentally. And when it gets tough, call me anytime. I love you." I could see a small tear in the corner of his eye. As hard as it was for me, it was harder for him to see me in my condition, a prisoner in a metal chair with wheels.

The therapist approached us with a skateboard, pushed aside the footrest for my left foot, and said, "Okay, you need to push up and back twenty times. Wave to me when you are done." That was easier than it looked.

The other exercises for my left leg included hip raises on a firm treatment couch and using my muscles to roll a ball back and forth while bending my knee.

For my right leg, we did the same exercise with the big ball. Nothing else. There was just too little bend in my right knee, and of course there was the added weight of the brace. The therapist was firm but gentle and did not push me when I reacted to the pain. At least not that day.

I felt like that old woman in front of my son. I was discouraged, and no amount of encouragement from David helped me feel better.

CHAPTER 13

REHAB, DAYS 3–4

The next two days passed with the same routine. Two therapy sessions, two two-hour CPM sessions. I also sent a hundred messages from my brain to my shattered right leg, with no response. I was determined to keep trying.

I felt more strength in my arms, and I was becoming an expert on the slide board. This added strength cut down on the time it took to make wheelchair trips.

The highlight of those two days was my first shower since the accident. My legs needed to be encased in plastic sleeves. Due to the pushing and pulling of getting the sleeves on and secured, it took an hour to get ready for just a ten-minute shower! But what a glorious ten minutes it was. I believe water is the best of God's gifts. Having a really clean body and being able to actually wash my hair was heavenly.

The counter to all this joy was my lack of progress on the CPM machine; 60 had gotten to be more bearable, but 65 was still torture.

I had nightly visits from Keith, as well as two or three calls each day. I also received calls from my staff, friends, family, and my grandchildren. The children asked if they could bring markers on Mother's Day to decorate my cast. Mother's Day, Sunday, May 13th, would make my 18th day in the hospital.

When Keith called Friday afternoon, he told me that the Executive Director from the Long Island Import Export Association had called to discuss my speech for the next week.

"She told me," he said, "that this meeting was geared to a mainly female audience and she asked me if you were in. Apparently, news of your accident did not reach her. When I told her where you were and what had happened, she was shocked and said that she would try to give you a call in the next few days. She asked if she should cancel the meeting? I told her no because I knew that you had already prepared your speech. Then I asked her if I could speak in your place, and she agreed saying that was a great idea. She thinks the women will love it. Are you okay with that?"

"Oh my God. I completely forgot about that. Yes, yes of course. You should do it. That would be great. I already did all the work."

"Where's your laptop?" he asked.

"Keith, my laptop is in my office. But let me explain what I wrote before you read it. I divided the presentation into two parts. The first part tells about how I got hired as an accountant by the owner of Dorf International and how I got into the freight forwarding business). The next part is the story of how we started Amber Worldwide. Barbara wanted me to highlight for the ladies how I grew our company to become the largest woman-owned freight forwarding company in the world."

"So," Keith teased, "did you include why they call you the Dragon Lady?"

"Well, I didn't tell them about the name specifically, but I did put in a few interesting challenges I had during my first trip to China in 1981. I thought it would add some color. You know, how I slept in a tent and lived on rice, tuna, and tea for three days after waiting two weeks for a visa. That I was the only woman on site, other than the middle-aged Chinese woman who was my interpreter, where they were loading garments on hangers into trucks for transport into Hong Kong. I left out the details about the rats at the airport and the primitive bathroom facilities. Why get them sick when they'll be eating?" I laughed.

"Hey, gotta go." I rushed. "One of the doctors just walked in. Bring the laptop when you come tonight, and we can go over it all. I love you. Bye."

Friday night, Delores and Shelly stopped in again on their way to dinner. They wanted to check that I was receiving good treatment from the hospital staff. Shelly's intervention had certainly helped a lot. I was grateful and told him so.

Keith came a bit later with flowers, and a teddy bear wearing a Get Well sweatshirt. Keith greeted me, with a smile.

"Hi, babe. Brought you this bear so you would have some company in bed." He hugged me gently and kissed me, and suddenly the tears came, deep and wet from the depths of my throat. The more I tried to stop, the more the tears and sobs continued.

"It'll be okay, babe," he soothed. My bruised chest still hurt, so he kept patting my back to soothe me, though I could feel him aching to hug me and make all the pain go away. Eventually the tears and sobs slowed. "Now, what brought all this on?" Keith asked.

"I miss you, Keith."

"But I'm right here, babe. Not to worry."

I pulled back a little and focused on him looking distraught, and whispered, "I miss sleeping with you, and feeling your body pressed into mine, and the touch of your arm cradling me. I miss our life, and our friends, and being able to feel the sun on my face, and breathing fresh air. Most of all, I miss our future." This was the first time I admitted aloud how scared I was. Big, brave, fearless me had suddenly vanished, and I was not quite sure what or who had taken her place.

Keith did not try to reassure me that everything was fine. He didn't say anything. He just kept holding me, and I calmed down. There was a comfortable silence between us.

He distracted me from my distress by bringing out my computer, so we could review some business and the contents of my speech that he would be delivering.

Even though I was basically bed-ridden, I needed to keep my mind working. Contributing my input on business issues kept me in touch with the world outside the hospital and rehab reality. I could make plans for the future and know I was still contributing. Strategizing, organizing, creating lists in my mind—working helped pass the time when I was doing monotonous exercises for my body.

Saturday morning, after my therapy, I returned to my room and began messaging my leg. After my fifth session, it finally happened! My right leg moved a little. Maybe an inch, but it moved. I needed to be sure I hadn't imagined it, so I concentrated really hard and repeated my little saying: "Brain to muscles... make my right leg move," and surprisingly, it DID! I was so excited I nearly fell out of the wheelchair. I started clapping my hands and congratulated my brain on a job well done.

There were a few more tries with success, then nothing. I told myself to give it a rest and try again later. I had such a feeling of pride and accomplishment. I was elated. Maybe, I said to myself, life could return to the way it was before April 24th.

Months later, I was up late watching a talk show and I saw Valerie Harper being interviewed. She had been diagnosed with an inoperable brain tumor, and the doctors had given her three months to live. Her interview took place six or seven months after her diagnosis. The host asked her to what she attributed her longevity beyond prognosis. Valerie responded that every day, many times during the day, she talked to her tumor. She said, "Listen up, tumor. You want to live, right? And if you want to live, that means I have to live, right? So, you need to stop growing, because if you continue to grow, I will die and if I die, so will you. It is in your best interest to keep the growth under control, so, behave!"

When I listened to her, I wondered how she came to the idea that she could get her brain to control her body. I knew I had done it and it made me smile. We were kindred spirits.

When Keith came early that Saturday afternoon, I told him the doctors had given me permission to go with him outside for Mother's Day. "You need to alert Mitch and David, set a time around lunchtime, and have them meet us outside. I am excused from one of my therapy sessions and the CPM morning torture. I have almost the whole day off!"

I instructed him that I wanted him to go to a sporting goods store and buy me a pair of basketball shorts in the men's department (they should fit over the brace) and a tee shirt of some kind. The weather report forecasted sunny and warm, with no rain.

I continued on with more good news. "The doctor was in this morning. He removed the last staple, the one that refused to come out. He said all was healing nicely and he planned to discharge me on Thursday. He did scold me as I am still only at 65 degrees, and he didn't want to let me go home, but I promised to keep working on the angle at home. He said he would prepare an order to the company that makes the CPM machine to deliver one to our home. They would also bring a portable commode and wheelchair, one that collapses to go in a car.

"A therapist will be coming to our house every other day to do exercises with me. That will help strengthen my left leg to the point I'll be able to use a walker, with my arms and one leg, to get around a little more easily. Of course, this can only happen after the ankle heals.

"In the first weeks, I will have a practical nurse with me for twenty-four hours. One daytime, one nighttime, beginning on Thursday night. A visiting nurse will come each day to monitor my vitals and give me the belly injection and take blood.

"Now," I continued, almost out of breath with excitement, "here comes the best part. I actually had my leg move! I was doing my messaging when it happened. I tested to be sure and it happened again. It moved about an inch. I don't know what excites me more, finally going home or having my leg move!"

And almost like an afterthought, I blurted, "And of course I will have my family all together on Mother's Day!" I was over the moon. I asked him not to say anything to the kids because I wanted to surprise them with my news myself.

The second I stopped talking, Keith was all over me with hugs and kisses and said, "I'm so proud of you, babe. Not to worry. We are going to lick this, I promise.

"I will take care of getting the house prepared for your home-coming. Josephine[1] will come to clean, and Gary[2] can help me move the furniture and rugs, so we can position a hospital bed, and the other things you will need, in the living room.

"On my way up to you, I bumped into the woman that drops in every once in a while from patient services, and she told me to wait for her, as she was going to stop by," Keith concluded.

With all my effervescing excitement, I thought this was a day I would never forget. I was on the way to getting my old life back!

---

[1] Long Beach Housekeeper.
[2] Elaine's nephew.

CHAPTER 14

MOTHER'S DAY

18 DAYS SINCE THE ACCIDENT

Mother's Day on May 13th dawned with a bright sun and hardly any wind moving the trees. I had completed all of the tasks required of me by the time Keith handed me a gorgeous bouquet of flowers and a bag with my new Mother's Day apparel. I donned a pair of men's black basketball shorts and coordinated white-and-black men's top with #18 embossed across the chest. The process of getting me into this new gear involved much twisting and turning while on the bed.

"Stunning!" Keith proclaimed as I rested back onto my pillows.

My darling husband knows me so well because he had brought my makeup bag, some perfume, and my wedding ring for this glorious celebration with my children. He said he would take the ring home again later, so it would not get lost.

Self-assessing after all the preparations on my face were completed, I declared, "Not bad." It helped my spirits so much to look at my old self in the mirror, even though my hair was totally unsettled, needed a cut, and my roots were showing.

"I'm ready to go out now. Are the kids here yet?"

"Yup," he answered. "They sent me a text about ten minutes ago."

I was so excited and happy that, for a few minutes, I forgot where I was. Having to slide down a board to get into the wheelchair quickly re-centered me.

As the doors opened to the real world, I asked Keith to stop for a moment. I wanted to take it all in. I closed my eyes. I got a whiff of pine from a large tree near the entrance and a floral ping from the spring flowers planted around the grounds. I felt the warmth of sun on my face. I listened to the birds singing and then… the best sound of all: grandchildren shouting, "Amah!" with glee.

Grandma, Nana, and Granny were names for old, gray-haired, chunky ladies who smelled of cold cream and spent their days baking cookies. That wasn't me. I was a corporate executive, who dressed in business suits and high heels, with impeccable makeup and smelled of expensive perfume. I was a world traveler, who hardly ever spent time in the kitchen, let alone baking cookies. When I asked my friends for alternatives to Grandma, I didn't find the right fit until my friend suggested the Chinese word for grandmother, Amah. That worked.

The grandkids came running and stopped short of the wheelchair.

"Will it hurt if I hug you?" Mitch's twelve year old daughter Jessica asked. Her brother Brent, ten years old, looked from me, to the cast, to the brace, and said nothing. David's nine year old daughter Ameerah ran around in back of me, put her arms around me, and kissed the back of my neck. I was positively glowing with happiness and pride.

"Where's Erica?" I asked.

Mitch responded, "Mom, we left her home. She had the sniffles and we didn't think it was wise for her to be here. And remember, she is only five years old and a little hard to handle. We'll bring her to see you once you get home."

"Promise?" I asked. "But have her call me."

"We brought indelible markers," Jessica said. "I want to be the first to draw a picture on your cast."

"Well, each of you should find a spot on the cast to decorate, so that there will be no fights. What do you say? Okay?"

Artwork progressed without conflict. Jessica just signed her name and wrote "I love you," substituting a heart for the word "love." Brent drew a teddy bear (or a reasonable facsimile of one) with "Get well" in his best printing, underneath the bear. And Ameerah just drew flowers of different colors wherever there was space not taken up by anything else. All in all, it was a VERY colorful and festive cast when they all completed their masterpieces.

The consensus was that I looked well, although much thinner and pale. Of course, there were many questions as this was the first time both my sons and their spouses had seen me since Easter. The questions came peppered at me equally from kids and adults. The most common question was "When are you coming home?"

I smiled and shared my great news. "I hope this week."

It surprised me how quickly I got tired. I guess Keith noticed it too and said, "I know you guys want to go for some lunch, and I think Amah needs to rest a bit. This is her first excursion out of the hospital, and she looks like she's beginning to fade."

"Before you go, I have something I need to show you," I interrupted. "You need to be very quiet, because I am sending a message to my leg from my brain. It's taken me a long time just to get my right leg to move a tiny bit, using a message I repeated hundreds of times. And finally, it did move yesterday. I am hoping I can show you what I can do."

It took a few minutes and then it happened. It actually did move, and they all saw it. They all applauded, and Mitch said it was just great. Somewhere, I have a family picture of all of us, taken by a passing visitor at the hospital. If I close my eyes, I can still see that photo and my face, showing the happiness I felt for just being alive.

Each of my family members hugged me more than once and kissed me too. The feeling of those little arms around my shoulders was something I cannot explain. The joy stayed with me throughout that day and the next. I think having that kind of joy to recall on demand helped me get through challenges that were yet to come.

The next few days passed in the same routines, as I counted down the hours until I would be discharged.

CHAPTER 15

LEAVING THE HOSPITAL

23 DAYS SINCE THE ACCIDENT

The rain on Thursday morning was heavy. Keith had arrived earlier with a suitcase to pack up all of my personal things. He brought a plastic poncho to cover me from the dark deluge I could see attacking my window.

Carol finished getting me into a pair of sweatpants.

"Time to go, young lady. Your husband is waiting downstairs and has told me that as soon as I get you into the ambulance, he will go on ahead so he can get the side door to your building opened for the attendant to wheel you inside, hopefully without you getting drenched."

As I looked around the austere room, my home for over two weeks, now stripped of anything that spoke of my personality or history, I felt a tiny bit of sadness. A little piece of me wanted to remain. This room was my haven. It afforded me security, protected me, and comforted me when things got bad. And of course, there was my steady companion, the clock. That clock got me through some brutal days.

At the same time, I also was quite delighted to be going home. Twenty-three days after my accident, I was given a large folder of instructions regarding home care and medications, and then there was nothing to do but wait for the ambulance driver to arrive.

A parade of staff wished me well and asked me to stop by and see them whenever I had appointments with doctors at the hospital, as I was wheeled down the hallway towards the exit lobby.

The overhang of the hospital entrance protected me from the weather while the driver opened the rear door of the ambulance. He positioned me onto the lift gate, strapped me into the chair, and then strapped the chair into the floor lock once I was securely positioned inside.

As we drove into the rain, the elation I had felt about leaving a few minutes earlier now turned to fear. The rain was so heavy and there was fog. It was like one of those movies where you know something horrible is going to happen because the ominous music fades in along with the fog, which conceals whatever terrorizes you.

What if there was an accident and I was strapped in and could not move? Maybe I would drown. I wanted to scream, "Take me back!" But I didn't. I closed my eyes. If I could not see where I was, then maybe I could cope? I could, however, still feel the motion, and although I tried to rationalize that I was not in a car, and that the driver was experienced, it did nothing to stop the terror.

Terror goes beyond fear. I had flashbacks, one after another. The sound of the crumbling metal, the jolt and then a thud as the car hit the ground, the repetition of my own screams from the iodine bath in the ER, the feeling of being all alone. Each bump in the road caused a large intake of breath and then the feeling of no breath at all, like being smothered. My fingers dug into the arms of the wheelchair so hard that my nails started to break. The driver was taking us down the road to the beach across a small isthmus of land, the Loop Parkway. The ocean was on both sides of the road. The ambulance swerved and I opened my eyes. I could see the water on both sides, with angry-looking waves crashing high. It seemed as if they were clawing at the land, hoping to get at me.

We made it home without incident. I whispered, "Thank you, God."

When Keith opened the door to our apartment, I was not facing my stylish and cozy living room, but hospital room number three. The sections of the couch were stacked upon one another in the corner. The rugs had been rolled up. A hospital bed was set up to face the television with a small table on one side and portable commode (the latest in chic living room styling?) on the other. The dreaded CPM machine was there on the floor, with the slide board on top of it. Another chapter was beginning. I doubted if my life would ever return to the way it had been before.

"Do you want something to eat or drink?" Keith asked.

"No. I'm tired. I just want to get into bed and take my pain meds."

I half listened to the visiting nurse when she arrived. I totally ignored the night nurse, except when I needed the bedpan.

I ate nothing and drank only a little water to get the meds down. I did not speak to anyone—not even Keith—for two days. I refused to get out of bed. I did not do any exercises. No CPM machine either. I told the therapist who came to help me move that I did not feel well and to come back in a few days. I was deep into depression and had fallen into a post-trauma sinkhole. The only thing I wanted were the painkillers. All the motivation and adrenaline I had in the hospital, pushing me to work hard in order to go home, had seemingly washed away on that rain-soaked drive back home.

CHAPTER 16

ACCLIMATING TO HOME

Keith came home from the office much earlier than usual on the second day I was home. He asked the aide, "Has she eaten anything?"

"No," she answered.

Keith told her to go home. I overheard him on the phone asking the night nurse to come a little later that evening.

He walked over to my bed and sat down facing me. I noticed that his blue eyes had turned steel gray as they connected with mine. I knew that meant he was angry.

Somehow compassion, anger, and a force of nature all combined in his words to me:

"You cannot give up. You have conquered the grief of losing your daughter and your parents. You made it through a nasty divorce. And together, we opened eight successful companies. It is out of character for you to give up! Just like you made your leg move, you'll find a way to get up and off that bed. To stand up and then walk!

"Remember the clairvoyant who told you about me and said I would be there with you for the rest of your life. I will support you and encourage you, and when it gets tough, I will give you the strength you need to succeed. You are the love of my life, and you cannot give up and leave me here on my own! I won't have it!"

Keith's speech left me no longer feeling sorry for myself but feeling sorry for him. During my recovery at the hospital and in rehab, and now during my self-pity party, I hadn't taken into account what Keith had been going through. He had been in the accident too. He had been physically hurt, not anywhere near as badly as I was, but my morose behavior had only heaped more hurt on him. For the most part, I had a good attitude, but not after coming home. I couldn't find the words for an apology, which in hindsight I should have made but didn't.

At the hospital, I hadn't sleep well. Aside from the nurses coming in ostensibly to check my vitals or administer medication every few hours (I was convinced they were just making sure I was still alive), I was awake devising a plan for how to resume my old life. I needed a pathway to getting on my feet, to partner with my brain to fool my leg into reaching the goal of the 90 degree angle, so that whenever my leg healed, I would be able to walk. But how? I was always looking at that clock on my bedside table and a plan came to mind like the ticking minute hand. Start the machine at 55 degrees, do three to five up and downs; then increase the angle one degree at a time, while increasing the number of bends with each degree. Then track the pain levels and adjust.

Now that I was home, I was going to put this plan into action. I was going to get back on my feet again, if not for myself, then for Keith.

Sitting up for any length of time was painful. I had lost most of the muscles in my rear end due to lack of movement. The rented hospital bed was not too comfortable. I found a special foam mattress and also a four-inch foam cushion for the wheelchair. These helped.

My stomach rebelled. Two days without eating or drinking anything except a little bit of water left me dehydrated and queasy. Even the soup that Keith fed me did not sit right.

On the morning after our bedside chat, Keith made sure I finished my soup and left me in the qualified hands of the aide as he left for work. I put my plan into effect. I was still on two oxycodone, every four to six hours. I knew that the optimum strength would be at 45 minutes after I took the tablet, and I knew that I had to be on the CPM machine two hours, twice a day. The machine had a dial to set the degree of bend, and I had reached 65 degrees without extraordinary pain before I left the hospital.

I programmed the home machine to 66 degrees and found it bearable. Taking it one degree at a time, I was able to reach 70 degrees before the pain was too intense. I returned to 65 degrees until the pain subsided and then went up one degree at a time again. When I again reached 70 degrees, I left it there for five minutes. I had a new clock in front of me, smaller than the hospital clock, but this one had an alarm. I put that to good use!

I followed the same procedure at night and was encouraged enough to reach 75 degrees! I congratulated myself and thought about combining this strategy with messaging my leg. I thanked my brain and body for their cooperation, and promptly decided to treat myself to a double helping of chocolate cake!

CHAPTER 17

First Post-Hospital Dr. Visit

27 Days Since the Accident

My appointment with Dr. Rotolo, the head of orthopedics at Nassau Medical Center, was on the fourth day after arriving home. I was to get x-rays, and he would report on my healing status. For this momentous appointment, I wanted to be clean. So, the night before my appointment, when Keith called to say he'd prepare the bathroom for my shower once he got home, I agreed willingly. He reminded the aide she could leave early and then signed off: "See you in a bit, darling."

This would be my second real shower since the accident. The first shower was an iodine bath of sorts, so that doesn't count; then I had the one unforgettable shower in the hospital, the one that required quite a production to cover all the parts of me that couldn't get wet. Now, I still had those challenges, but I wasn't in a hospital room made specifically to be wheelchair-accessible. This was going to be interesting.

My wheelchair, narrow as it was, did not fit through the door to our bathroom. Keith wheeled me back down the hall to wait while he took the bathroom door off the hinges. Let's try this again…

This time, we used the crank to keep reducing the width of the adjustable wheelchair until Keith was finally able to back me into the bathroom. All I could do was laugh at the ridiculousness of the situation. I told him we needed to hang a sign in the hallway to warn visitors that someone was using the bathroom, as there was no longer a door. I proposed using a bathroom pass on a hook like we had in my elementary school. No pass, no passage!

Backwards was the only way in for me. The chair was right up against the sink, and there was perhaps five inches to spare from my knees to the opposite wall. First hurdle overcome.

The second hurdle was mere moments afterwards. We both realized at the same time that trying to get the protective vinyl covering on my legs (to protect them against water damage) necessitated yet another trip back down the hallway.

An hour later, after a lot of tugging and pushing, I was ready for the transfer to the shower seat. The arms of the wheelchair had been removed. I was able to use the slide board to shimmy down to the shower seat. From there, I was able to pull my left foot inside the tub while my right leg gingerly rested on the edge of the top of the tub. All of this production, for a shower that took less than ten minutes.

Needless to say, showers became a very irregular event. However, this was the first time I could remember laughing since I had come home. And as I look back, I don't think I laughed heartily at all during my twenty-three days in the hospital.

On the day of the appointment, I was in decent spirits. I had showered the night before and had a great session on the CPM in the morning. I was able to eat lunch and prepared to go to the doctor. All I had to do was to be able to get into the car. Another hurdle. But this turned out to be more than just a logistical challenge.

Our rental car was a four-door Chrysler sedan. It had a front passenger seat that could be moved all the way back, until it touched the rear seat. The door had a wide angle opening. It wasn't hard for me to transfer myself from the wheelchair to the car, as the hospital had given me lots of training with a mock car. So, off we went.

Keith drove very slowly even though there was hardly any traffic. Whenever any car came too close, or if he needed to step on the brake with pressure, I took a huge intake of air and a prayer that nothing bad would happen. Relief came when we finally arrived at Dr. Rotolo's office. If I could have skipped away from that car with relief to have arrived, I would have!

I had several x-rays taken of both legs, and then we were ushered into the doctor's office. "Well," he said, "I have good news and some not so good. Your ankle is nearly completely healed; we will remove the cast today and put on a brace. I am making arrangements for a physical therapist to come to your home. She'll get you up on your left leg and teach you the exercises to help strengthen your ankle. In a short time, you'll be able to get around with a walker." This was great news. Independence was a tantalizing thought.

"As you know, the damage to your right femur was extensive. A comparison of the hospital x-rays, with the ones we just took, show no healing of the bone at all." I was surprised but he continued before I could ask questions. "I can't tell you why at this time. A technician will come to your house tomorrow and take measurements for an electromagnetic device that you must wear ten hours a day. Hopefully, this will cause the bone to start the healing process. It does have a battery but, for the most part, it needs to be plugged in while it's on. I prefer that you do two five-hour sessions, but you can do three sessions, as long as each session is at least two hours. And it is not to be worn while you are sleeping. When you come back to see me in a couple of weeks, we'll see if there is any improvement. In the meantime, I am putting you on an antibiotic, in case there is some infection that the bloodwork does not show.

"Your insurance company needs to approve this treatment and the cost. If they do not, you will need to pay for it yourself. It is necessary. Hopefully, by using it, the holes will start to fill in. Unfortunately, it is quite expensive. $5,000." He repeated, "It is my hope that the stimulation will start the process of filling in the holes in your bone."

Keith and I just looked at each other, surprised at the price but knowing we had no choice and would pay if the insurance company rejected this treatment.

The next part of our visit was the physical exam. Dr. Rotolo had me get onto the examination table with my legs straight out in front of me. In all the many days since the accident, I had avoided looking at my leg. I had never seen it without the brace. It would have been impossible for me to have ever imagined what I now saw. It wasn't the scar, which was still an angry red but not so wide; it was the way my whole leg had shrunk down to nothing! The skin was hanging off the bone, and there were several wide patches of discoloration. Only my toes were a normal size. The thigh had been covered with a thin layer of gauze and was now totally exposed. The muscles had almost completely disappeared. It truly made me physically ill to look at it.

Use it or lose it was all I could think of. The doctor took in all of my shriveled body as matter of fact. I looked over to where Keith had been sitting and was now standing, looking at my leg and just shaking his head. I guess tears were cascading down my face, because the doctor, seeming to find some compassion, took my hand and said, "Don't worry. Once you start your strength training exercises, the muscle tone will improve."

He went on to critique aloud what he was seeing. "I do see that you are getting a better bend out of the knee. Once you can get to 90 degrees, you will have formed a right angle with your leg, and this is what you need to be able to walk the way you did before.

"But, no matter what," he continued in a very ominous, serious tone, "you need to remember that at no time can you EVER put any weight on that right foot, as there would be a good chance for the bone to shatter further. So, you need to be very careful as you get up that you put your weight on that left foot and ankle. Be sure you have your balance whenever you get up. Believe me, in a short time, you'll be able to use the walker, your arms, and your left leg to get around. Keep up with your arm exercises. When you are at least partially ambulatory, you'll feel better. Not just physically, but mentally as well. You are in excellent health, considering your age."

Seeing the defeated look on my face, Dr. Rotolo added, "In a very short time, with exercise and putting the weight on it, your left leg, will return to normal. I'll give you some topical medication to fade the scars; it can be used on both legs. Remember, there are eight screws in a metal plate, and that is ALL that is holding your bone together!

"I'm also giving you a prescription for outside physical therapy, to be started once you have regained some strength in your left leg. You can take the brace off your right leg only when you get to 90 degrees on the CPM machine. We have measured the degree on your leg. I'm disappointed that you're not yet at 90 degrees. You need to push it."

The ride home was as distressing as the ride there, especially after hearing the bad news. My decision was to follow my daily plan to reach 90 degrees, as it was working, and also to do the best I could with the physical therapy. I would continue sending the mental message to my leg to move; I could now lift my leg six inches off the footrest.

I looked forward to getting up on at least one leg and training to use a walker, which would allow me more freedom in the apartment and easier access to the pure pleasure of a shower—and also to getting out of the house to go to physical therapy at Long Beach Hospital. I called LBH as soon as I got home, and they accepted me and set up an appointment.

The next morning, I contacted our car insurance company and advised them of the cost of the new device as well as what the doctor thought it could accomplish and asked if I was covered. The agent put me on hold as she pulled my file. She advised me that I had already reached the medical limit on the policy, which was $50,000. I was amazed at how quickly the limit had been met since medical insurance had covered many of the medical expenses, so that $50,000 was covering our deductibles and co-pays. I had never seen any of the bills, and Keith never spoke of them to me.

"What happens now?" I asked her.

Her reply was a question. "Do you have other coverage?"

"Medicare and private health insurance," I responded.

"No, that's not what I'm asking. Do you have other vehicles covered with another company? If you do, then you need to contact them as soon as possible. You have coverage with them for the amount provided in that policy. Be sure to verify the amount with them."

Keith's car was the SUV he was driving on the day of the accident. It had been purchased and registered in Florida when we opened the Miami office, and that was why his insurance carrier was not the same as mine. My car was registered and insured in New York.

Apparently, according to this woman, if an older person on Medicare is in a car accident, then it is the responsibility of the car insurance company to be billed for the medical treatment and not Medicare. To help us process all this, she offered, "I will send you a letter advising you that the payout for your medical bills has now been fulfilled to the limit of the policy. The other carrier will require this in addition to the other paperwork. But you are covered. Trust me on that. We'll send letters out to companies, doctors, and any healthcare providers who send us an invoice in the future, explaining that we are no longer responsible for payment, and you'll be getting a copy of that letter. Those invoices will undoubtedly be sent to you until the other carrier takes over." The very helpful customer service person gave me her name and employee number and said I should call if there was anything else I required at any time. She then wished me the best of luck and a speedy recovery.

Fortunately, Keith and I had the money. Our companies were profitable. I didn't have to worry about being able to pay. However, like everyone else who pays for insurance year after year, I'd rather have them pay than me! I made a note to contact the insurance agent who handled our medical insurance for the office and to contact Keith's car insurance company.

As soon as I hung up from that call, the technician that was to do the fitting for the electromagnetic machine called and said he would come in the late afternoon. The health aide had come and started to prepare breakfast. I called Keith at the office to advise him about what his auto insurance company rep had told me. I asked him to contact the insurer of my car and find out what was needed to start the claim with them.

"Don't forget," I said, "you need to give them the information on Dr. Rotolo and to stress that the technician will be here this afternoon, and we need to start the ball rolling to get that device." I knew he had all the paperwork on the company that was to provide the device, and I reminded him that our controller had a copy of my auto insurance policy in a file in his office.

CHAPTER 18

DEAR MOM, DEAR GOD

May 20th was my mother's birthday. She had passed away several years prior. I silently wished her a happy birthday. I then asked her if she could ask God to continue to provide me with the strength I needed to do whatever was necessary to get up out of my chair and stand on my own two feet and walk again. Perhaps my mother could accomplish this on my behalf?

This was the first time since the accident that God had entered my thoughts. I was not a religious person in terms of prayers or asking for help or blaming God for my misfortunes. To this day, I have never thrown up my arms yelling at God, *why me?* Not when my daughter died, not when I went through the divorce from my first husband. Not even after the accident. It was not that I blindly accepted my fate. It was more that I accepted the trials, and somehow deep down, I knew that I would find the strength. Or perhaps that it would somehow be provided.

But this time was different. The accident left me physically damaged in addition to the emotional trauma. I was old, not just older. Seventy. My body was seventy. The Bible says three score and ten. I questioned whether this was another trial or had I some-how cheated death? And if it was another trial, what did God expect me to do? What tools would God provide, if any? Would they all come from me? From my connection to my brain, I wondered? Or from the sheer determination to get me up and out of that chair? All these thoughts came rapid-fire into my mind.

STOP IT, I commanded myself. *Just stop it.* I motivated myself to stay positive, concentrate, get on with my exercises, keep push-ing, and to hit the 90-degree mark that was my first goal.

I called out to the aide to bring me the pain medication, and I set the alarm for thirty minutes so the aide could help me set up the CPM machine. In the meantime, I continued the messaging from my brain to my leg, observing the positive results. I could now lift my leg even higher, and soon, I knew, reviewing my progress, I would be able to lift it parallel to the cushion.

In the early afternoon, a young man came with the electromagnetic device that was supposed to heal my bones. He adjusted the fitting and showed me where I needed to position it and how to work the controls. I couldn't feel anything except a little bit of heat.

He handed me a copy of the invoice and said he had been advised that I was covered under my auto insurance policy. I signed the section that acknowledged that the cost was mine to bear if the insurance did not pay for it. He added my credit card number to the agreement, winking at me, and explained, "I just need to do this in case you intend to run away."

When Keith came home, he brought some papers from my insurance company for me to sign. He said it was no problem and that they would be taking over the payments. In the file he carried was their contact numbers and copies of relevant paperwork.

Lisa, the in-home therapist arrived at 6:00 p.m. Lisa had long brown hair tied back in a ponytail, and wore a polo shirt and athletic pants. She looked very young, but she was thorough. She asked me a lot of questions, especially about the in-hospital physical therapy.

"Do you have a pair of older sneakers that perhaps are a bit stretched out? I'll need the left one and a sock. You're going to stand up on your left foot. I will be here on one side and your husband on the other. You may experience some pins and needles and maybe a little pain, or maybe none of that at all. Remember, that foot hasn't had any weight on it for almost a month. To ensure that your right leg won't be able to touch the floor, under doctor's instructions, I'm going to slightly change the angle of the brace." And Lisa set about organizing the therapy space and leg brace.

It felt strange to have something more than a sock on my foot. There was a little trouble getting my foot into that sneaker, even though most of the laces had been loosened to allow for the swelling.

Lisa told me to relax (as if I could) as she applied the brake on the wheelchair. She pulled out the footrests and removed the armrests.

"Now," she said, "before we pull you up, put your arms on the cushion and as we are lifting, you push hard with your arms. On the count of three, up you go." And there I was, standing on one foot, just like a crane. "Well done," she said.

My leg started shaking, my muscles rebelling. "Bend your leg. You remember how to sit, don't you?" she asked. And down I went, out of breath but exhilarated!

"Okay, great! Now I'll get on with the therapy, which will help you gain strength in your left leg, and you'll learn how to use your arms so you can stand up and use the walker. I'll leave you with some exercises for your legs that you can do in bed and two sets of hand weights for your arms." Lisa emphasized that she would reappear every day that week at about the same time, and she would need Keith to be here to assist me in getting up. She then comforted me, saying, "You'll see, in a short time the shaking will stop." And then, "I know you'll be starting physical therapy at Long Beach Hospital next week. I know the guys there, and you have made an excellent choice."

And thus, the next phase of my recovery and journey back to the old me had begun. It was twenty-eight days since the accident. I had every confidence that the device would do its job and the process of healing would begin. All I needed to do was my part.

The second try to get me up on my feet the next day was easier. I was shaking less and my fear of getting up was diminishing.

Strangely, after a few days of putting weight on my left foot, the sole of my foot began to peel. The therapist explained that I might start to grow calluses on that foot due to the extreme pressure of my weight on it.

CHAPTER 19

A NEW KIND OF WORK SCHEDULE

May in New York is always a spectacular month. The weather is perfect. The air is warm and dry. Spring flowers, trees, and bushes are in bloom, and their fragrances fill the air. The colors are not to be believed. Living on the beach, being able to see the Atlantic Ocean's waves and watch the changing color of the water, helped remind me that I was glad to be alive. But while the doctor had not put any restrictions on going outside, I was not yet ready.

It wasn't easy to adjust to being home. In that first week, there were more downsides than upsides. I couldn't be left alone. At least in the hospital, I had a private room all to myself. Now I had one aide with me from around 8:30 a.m. until 4:30 p.m. The next one came for the night shift from 8:00 p.m. to 8:00 a.m. the next morning. Keith was with me from 5:00 p.m. until morning.

The visiting nurse came daily, around the time the first aide left, to check my vitals and give me an injection into my belly. She didn't know that I had learned how to do this in the hospital already. Like then, the heparin injection was to prevent blood clots from forming as I was virtually inactive. The nurse taught me how to keep a daily tracking sheet, which included taking my temperature twice daily at specified times, how many times I went to the bathroom, how much water I had to drink, if I was eating or not, my sleep pattern, and the number oxycodone I was taking and when.

My schedule went something like this: Waking up around 6:00 a.m. I used the early morning hours to put the electromagnetic device on. I had to do that for five hours, twice a day. Then, when the aide came in, it was a sponge bath, breakfast, pain meds, and two hours on the CPM machine to move my knee. Then back with the other device for three hours; then exercises and lunch. I saved the other time with the CPM machine for evening.

It was hard for me to sit for any length of time, so I saved my time in the wheelchair for afternoons when I would focus on work-related tasks at the dining room table. I had to finish the contract for the sale of our London company.

Additionally, I had visits from neighbors and friends. Most people were considerate enough to check in by phone first. This was important to me as the portable commode was next to my bed in the living room, and advanced notice gave my aide time to cover it and move it to the terrace before the guest arrived.

It was wonderful to see everyone but also tiring. I found myself repeating the same responses over and over again to the same questions about the details of the accident. Now, looking back, I sometimes wonder if the repetition is why all of the details of the first two days after the accident are indelibly etched into my brain. The visits gave me a diversion from my routine, and the hugs were a definite benefit. We humans need the physical contact of other human beings. Each hug seemed to transmit strength. I could actually feel the energy going inside me along with the caring of the giver.

Keith would normally get home between five and five thirty and spend some time with me. We'd have dinner together, while he informed me of what had transpired in the office that day. We would wait together for Lisa to arrive.

Within a few days of being home, I was able to set my routine and once set, I programmed the clock and my phone with alarms and reminders. My clock was always dependable, always my friend, and (besides Keith) was the only constant in my life since the accident. The clock was the governor of my daily life.

CHAPTER 20

LONG BEACH HOSPITAL

My next trip out since being home was traveling in the car to Long Beach Hospital for my first outside physical therapy. This time, the car ride was easier than I thought it would have been. Maybe that's because, since LBH was only two miles away, we could drive slowly and avoid highways.

I had confidence in LBH rehab, no doubt because it was in a hospital. The angle of my right leg was now at a consistent 80 degrees. My body had responded very positively to all the exercises. I had real muscles in my arms and, as a side bonus, the ever-sagging flesh underneath my arms (attributed to normal aging) had greatly diminished. My left leg had improved too. The one area that did not improve was my midsection; and whereas it had been firm before the accident, it was no longer so. And truthfully, it still isn't, so thank God for Spanx!

Two young men approached us as Keith and I entered the physical therapy room.

"Hi. I'm Davie, and this is Ron. Who are you?" He sounded, and kind of looked like, the Cheshire Cat in Disney's animated version of *Alice in Wonderland*. His big, wide grin showed all of his teeth; he only lacked the stripes.

"I'm Elaine. I have an appointment today at 2:00 p.m. to start my physical therapy, here in the hospital. I gave all of my information to the nice young lady who answered the phone yesterday."

Davie shared that I would regrettably still have paperwork to complete as he collected my driver's license, social security card, and insurance information. I also gave him the car insurance information to make sure they were the ones to be invoiced.

As Davie looked over the script from my doctor, he said, "I'm the therapist assigned to your case. And Ron here, he'll take over when I'm not around. But today, you lucky person, you will have both of us." I was treated to another Cheshire smile as he looked up from the paperwork.

Paperwork out of the way, I was wheeled into a private room and transferred to an exercise table. Keith asked if it was okay for him to stay and was assured that it was fine.

They began with a measurement of the angle of my right leg. Next was the testing of my left ankle and its rotation, followed by some kind of strength test on my left leg. Davie asked about the exercises I did in the trauma hospital and what I had been doing at home with Lisa. I answered fully, and then also told him about the electromagnetic machine and the CPM daily workouts.

"We are going into the main room, where I'll have you transfer yourself to one of the beds. We want to see how you manage with the slide board. Notice that these beds are about the same height as your bed at home. Beds are easier than chairs to get in and out of, unless the chairs have arms. I am going to show you how to get up from that height using a walker.

"Learning to take steps with the walker is lesson number two," he continued, "when I see you again tomorrow. Your left leg and your arms are strong enough to do this. I am well aware that at no time can you put any weight on your right leg. Trust me, you do have the strength. Ron and I will be holding onto you.

"Before you start any training, you'll need to do some breathing exercises. These help in many ways. First of all, you will be filling up your lungs with air, oxygen; this helps a bit with pain. They are also meant to relax you and, in so doing, diminish some of the initial fear you will have."

They placed a walker in front of where I was seated on the bed and had me put my hands flat on the bed on either side of me. Ron had a walker in front of him. He was sitting on the bed opposite me and said, "Now watch me." He rocked back and forth, raising his butt a little with each rock, while his hands remained on the bed. "After you're comfortable rocking, keeping your hands on the bed—probably only your fingertips will remain on the bed— and use the strength in your left leg to get you to stand up on that one leg. If you lose balance, all you need to do is flatten out your hands while lowering yourself back to the bed."

Making sure I was nodding to indicate I understood what he was explaining, Ron continued with final instructions: "Make sure that the back of your left leg is touching the bed. At all times you need to be aware of that right leg. Due to the position of the brace, it will always be slightly in front of you and, of course, at that position, off the floor. So, let's try it. One of us will be on the bed with you and the other, when you are ready to stand, will support you under your arm. We need for you to see where the walker is in relation to your feet and body.

"Once you're standing and sure of your balance, you will need to take one of your hands and put it on the walker. And then the other. Notice the tennis balls on two of the feet of the walker; this is for stability. Okay, now, let's rock…"

Davie looked at my face, and maybe also at Keith, who looked more nervous than I did, and asked, "How do you feel? Are you comfortable? Confident? Ready to stand up?"

"Yup," I answered.

"Don't grab the walker until you have your balance; this could make you fall. If you're unsteady, you'll just go backwards onto the bed. Soft landing, kid, just like on the moon. Are you scared?"

I shook my head no.

"Not even a little? No? You're a liar, but you have guts, I'll give you that," Davie laughed. "Remember, Ron has you and I am next to you on the bed. No chance here for any mishaps. Start the rocking, and now you go up."

A few rock-a-billys later and I was up on one foot, holding onto the walker.

"You did great!" they said in unison. There I was… up on my own power! It was more thrilling than when I had gotten up on my own foot the first time. Was that really only a week before? I knew this time I did it under my own power. Their hands were on my body only as a safety net.

"Now you need to learn how to sit down. Never, never go to sit unless you can feel the back of your legs touching a bed or chair. Reach back with one hand till you find the bed. It's okay for the other to hold onto the walker as you ease yourself down. And keep that right leg out a bit as you do it. *Comprende? Si?*"

Davie was right. I really had been scared to death, but I was more scared of remaining in that chair for the rest of my life. Now at least I was learning how to get around, if only a little, and I could dream of having a rear end again. Mine was currently as flat as a pancake.

There was no pain, only discomfort, and very little shaking. The two oxycodone I had taken before leaving the house were doing their job.

"Now, on to the good part," Davie said. "Your exercises."

These were more strenuous and had more repetitions than the ones in the hospital, and some were very different. The session was about an hour, and I was exhausted at the end. I was also pleasantly surprised at how much strength I had in my arms and my one good leg. My left leg did shake, but never so much as the first time it had borne all my weight, the week before.

I knew that once I got home, when the painkillers left my body and the ice pack melted, I would be staring at the clock and counting down the minutes until I could pop the next pills.

My dependency on oxycodone was growing, but I needed the drugs to help me get over my fears and to deal with the pain. That morning, I set up a plan to cure myself of my pain pill addiction. My plan would go into effect the day after I hit 90 degrees on the CPM machine. There was no doubt in my mind that I had the will and the skill to do it.

At the end of the session, as Keith and I were leaving LBH, he said, "I haven't enough words to tell you how proud of you I am. How much I love you. And next week, I am registering you for the Olympics!" This not only made me laugh, but also a blush crept up onto my cheeks.

I hope that everyone else out there who goes through something life-changing has the kind of support I had from my husband. I'm not sure if I would have been as tough and motivated if I didn't want so badly to get back to our life together.

The cell phone rang just as we were getting home. It was Mitch calling to see how everything went.

"Hey, Mom," he said. "I have a thought. I think you can do without the night nurse. You and Keith have cell phones, and you have your house phone too. So, what I thought was that you really only need someone with you when you have to use the potty, right? And if you're not using the bedpan—or even if you are, Keith can handle that. No poops at night, right? Maybe on the weekend, give your nurse a couple of nights off and see how it works. And keep the bear with you for company at night."

My son had given me a teddy bear about the size of a three-month-old baby, back when he came to see me during the first week at the hospital when I was lost in Never Neverland. It was the color of a lion cub with soft, plush, velvet fur, and had big brown eyes. A red ribbon was tied festively around his neck that said, "I love you. Get well soon." I don't know what it is about teddy bears and the comfort they bring. I had the little one Keith had brought me, and it sat next to its big brother, Mitch's bear. These bears had been perched on the windowsill, smiling at me, in both hospital rooms I had been in.

CHAPTER 21

THINKING TOO MUCH?

Keith and I tried out Mitch's night schedule idea using the house and cell phones. It was a more challenging transition for Keith than me. Our businesses had offices all over the globe, and while normally Keith could just turn off the phone at night so we wouldn't be disturbed, with the possibility that the call could be me needing him, he wound up answering business calls all night too. Eventually, we figured out how to differentiate the calls. I think Keith was worried about me calling and him not answering. I know he was taking his frustration and anger out on me when the phone wouldn't stop ringing.

A month after we started this "no night nurse" routine, I overheard him telling a friend about our trials during the first weeks at home. "Worst thing ever, that suggestion from Mitch to use our house and cell phones and letting the night nurse go! I grew to hate the ring of my phone. So much so, I was tempted to throw the phone into the ocean. After a few nights of torture, I was talking to Pratik, my ops manager, who is very phone savvy, and he told me he could set up my phone so that there were two different ringtones.

I kept the old ring for Elaine and remembered, once in the house, to keep the phone on vibrate. And just before I went to bed, I put the ringer back on. I knew no one except Elaine would call me late at night. My only worry was that if she discovered what I had done, she might think I was having an affair. You know I would never do that."

As for me, not wanting to disturb my husband more than absolutely necessary, I often waited until the last minute before I made the potty call. Afraid I might have an accident, I told the daytime aide where I had some old Kotex pads and hid one under my pillow. When Keith went to bed, I positioned it between my legs, held together by my crossed thighs, just in case. I was well past the age of needing it for its original purpose. I slept flat on my back and didn't move all night because of the brace on my leg, so the pad stayed secure.

This was the price we paid for some privacy. And this was how I realized we each protected the other.

Life had become about endurance. Continuance may be the operative word. It was not life as it had been for me, nor for Keith. His daily salvation was going to the office to get a break from caregiving. Nothing about the way I was living resembled my life before the accident.

I started to resent it. "It" being life. I remind myself, "Be glad you are alive," but I questioned: If this was living, did I really want to live? And why was I alive, when I should have been dead? What had the great almighty God planned for me? Had I not already gone through enough? Or was I here only for Keith, to appease the guilt I knew he felt for being the driver of the car that put us both in this position? Sometimes, I could quickly push these negative thoughts away. Some days I admit I probably wasn't the most charming company, for anyone!

When I shared with my friend Jill how I was feeling, she said, "Okay, let's have a party!"

"A party?" What was she talking about?

"Yeah. Just us girls. Like in the old days. A pajama party!" And she was into planning mode. "Let's pretend we are teenagers. I can get us lots of CDs from the fifties and sixties. We can order in pizza and beer and even vodka too. And—" since she knew I was on drugs and couldn't drink, "—you can smell the alcohol. I'm gonna call the girls and get them to come tomorrow night. Tell Keith he can go out and that you'll have five babysitters." Jill ended her plan with a nod of conviction. And so, it was executed.

Jill bought white shorts and tee shirts for all of us and helped me change. We were six women transported back decades into our youth.

"Okay, listen up," Jill said. "This tarp has to cover the floor and we need to cover Elaine's chair in plastic. See this bag?" She held up a plastic sack from Michael's Art Supplies and then pulled out a hat. "It has body markers and body paint. All washable. Take a number from the hat." We all did. "On the label of your tee shirt is a number. That number represents the body you will be painting. All of your drawings must be x-rated. But not super graphic. *Well, not graphic enough to get you arrested.*"

We laughed and laughed and joked about the theme of the artwork. Scandalous!

Jill continued, "You have one hour to complete the painting. Then we eat. And then... Well, I will tell you after we eat," she teased.

We began our painting projects while the girls all drank and sang along to the music. We reminisced about each song playing. After an hour, my face hurt from smiling and laughing so much. When we were done, each of us was covered head to toe in paint.

"Okay, everybody, now it's potty time, not party time." We all followed Jill's instruction. When we were all back in the living room, Jill opened the door and said, "Okay, everybody out. We are going to have a live art show outside."

After we got over our initial reticence (my friends with the help of alcohol), oh my God! What a gas it was. The neighbors on the street loved it more than we did. Back upstairs my friends showered off but not before many pictures were taken.

"You," Jill said, "must remain painted till Keith gets home."

When Keith came in, his first reaction was shock, and then he had a fit of hysterical laughter.

"Well, we must be going," Jill said conspiratorially, "but now you can treat Elaine to an x-rated shower. And don't forget, we want a full shower report in the morning!" She laughed and started pushing my friends out of the apartment.

I thanked them all and said, "This was the best medicine ever. I will look at these pictures and remember and laugh. Thanks again. I love you all."

As May turned to June, the warmer and longer days of summer allowed for respite from the boredom of my routine: ten hours a day on the electromagnetic device, four hours a day on the CPM machine, one hour of home exercise daily, physical therapy three times a week at the hospital, and a few hours of drug-induced sleep.

With more daylight hours, I looked forward to late afternoons when Keith would wheel me over to the mini boardwalk near our home, so I could be at the beach and watch the waves. Welcome visits from friends and neighbors occasionally led to dinners out in restaurants. I treasured these pieces of normalcy, but they came at a price. The fatigue afterward was challenging.

Thank goodness for FaceTime. I was able to stay in touch with my grandchildren. Not the same as having them with me, but a good thing considering my limited ability to travel and to get around.

The first fear I needed to deal with was being in the car again, and the second was my inability to hold my water for more than four hours (along with the complications of evacuating my system).

Whenever Keith and I got in the car to go anywhere, he would be nervous because I was still riddled with anxiety. I would uncontrollably gasp large intakes of breath any time Keith hit a hard brake or executed a sharp movement.

"Stop that," he would say. But I couldn't.

I always answered Keith, "I cannot help it. It's an auto reflex." And he would get angrier and angrier.

I never traveled with my eyes open. I was like a child hiding under the covers for protection from ghosts. If I had my eyes closed, if I could not see the road, I would not be afraid. It did help, but only a little.

Now and again, in my head I would blame my husband for my current state of being. It was an accident, right? But was it? There was no traffic that day. It had been clear and the road was dry. Was he not paying attention? He had a habit of spitting out the window, turning his head to do so. He told me he had heard something and then the car changed direction. He said he was in the right lane, but he never drove in the right lane. Sometimes, I would reason I was being unfair, and I would mentally self-correct. And then there were other times, though not too many, when I would not.

CHAPTER 22

ONLY ONE STEP

3 MONTHS SINCE THE ACCIDENT

As much as I was getting stronger and more confident when I was up and moving about using the walker, there was the ever-present anxiety of losing my balance and having my right leg hit the floor. The aide was always behind me on the trips down the hall to the bathroom. The hallway was too narrow for her to walk next to me.

And then, on July 8th, just as I was coming down the hallway, it happened. Somehow, I misjudged the corner molding. I lost my balance, and my right foot hit the floor. The corner actually saved me as I was able to lean against it. Even though the aide was right there, there was nothing she could do except to grab onto me. I started screaming in panic, "Oh my God, oh my God, I can't believe I did this!" I kept repeating, "Call Keith! Call Keith! He needs to come home!"

Annie, my aide, had her arm around me. "I gotcha, I gotcha" she repeated soothingly. She was somehow able to drag me on my one leg over to the wheelchair and sat me in it.

"Deep breaths, Elaine. Take some deep breaths," Annie instructed. "I'll call Keith and then I'm calling the doctor."

My mind was racing. *Oh God! What if they can't save my leg? What if it has shattered more? What if they have to cut it off?* Not that I was getting too dramatic or anything!

I was in full-on panic mode. All that work. All those months potentially wasted. My crying was uncontrollable as the panic set further in.

I remember how calm Annie was, and with her demeanor as example, I was able to regain my composure. I heard her speaking into the phone: "This is Annie, Mrs. Rosendorf's aide. She lost her balance and her bad leg hit the floor… No! I don't think it was anything more than a tap… We need to come right over? Her husband is on his way home."

Nancy, the doctor's assistant, was on the other end of the line when Annie handed me the phone. Nancy said, "The doctor is here, and he'll see you whenever you get here. From what I have been told, the probability is that there has been no damage. Try to keep your leg elevated."

Twenty minutes later, Keith arrived at the apartment. He and Annie got me into the back seat of the Chrysler. My legs were stretched out in front of me. Annie put two pillows under my right leg. Fifteen minutes later, we were at the doctor's office. They literally dragged me off the back seat and slid me into the wheelchair. Keith told Annie to take me up while he parked the car.

I was calmer and more in control of myself by the time we reached the doctor's office. On the trip over, I wasn't preoccupied by my fear of being in a car. I never took my eyes off my watch, which was how I knew it was exactly a fifteen-minute drive. The watch kept me calm. As the minute hand went around, I kept repeating in my head: *It only touched the floor. No weight was really on it. Therefore, no damage is likely.* The pace of the repetition was controlled by the second hand. My watch, like the clock in the hospital, was my savior once again.

At the reception desk, Annie told the young lady to get Nancy; they were expecting us. Nancy took me immediately to x-ray. Once the pictures were taken, she wheeled me to an examination room where Keith was waiting. When he saw my face, he shook his head and soothed, "Please, babe, try to stay calm and try not to worry."

Easier said than done, I thought. And my mind continued with self-criticism. *I was always so careful. Maybe I was overconfident? Too sure of myself?*

Nancy soon knocked, opened the door, and let us know that Dr. Rotolo would arrive in a few minutes.

Smiling, Dr. Rotolo entered the room holding my x-rays. "The good news is that the x-rays compared to those taken in the hospital show that your touchdown was exactly that… just a touchdown."

"What a relief!" I sighed as my entire body relaxed. I hadn't realized how tensed up I was until the tension left.

"That's the good news. Sorry, Elaine. It's not all good. The x-ray shows that there is still no healing."

"None?" I questioned, as a deep sadness entered my soul.

"Could be a lot of reasons why," he said.

"Like what?"

"Well, there could be a low-grade infection, which the blood tests are unable to pick up. There could be no connection from the capillaries to the bone tissue, which sometimes occurs when there is extensive damage like yours. And I don't like to say it, but your age could be a major factor."

"How can you find out the cause?"

"The only way to find out would be to operate, which I'm not in favor of at the moment. My plan is to continue the program you are on for another two weeks. Sometimes it just takes longer for the electromagnetic device to stimulate the bone and for the body to react. And truthfully, at your age, we would anticipate a longer time for healing."

I interrupted, "But my ankle healed up fine. Worst case, what can you do if in another two weeks there's still no change?"

"I am considering doing a bone graft."

"What's that?"

"We can take some bone from your pelvis or bone that is donated by a cadaver and grind it up, add some artificial bone and antibiotics, and plaster up the holes. And see if there's any sign of infection. But let's not jump the gun until I see you in two weeks. See the receptionist on the way out. And TRY to get some rest."

There I was, teaming with mixed emotions. Ten minutes was all the time I had between the high of finding out there was no damage, to the terrible low of knowing there had been no healing.

No words passed from anyone's lips in the car on the ride home. Annie, Keith, and I were all in our own minds. Once upstairs, Annie got me into the hospital bed. Keith had gone to park the car. Annie asked if she could get me anything, and I just motioned to my medicines.

Other than my first two days home after the accident, I think this was the first time I could unequivocally admit to being depressed. Had all my efforts been in vain? I had forced myself, even in the worst of times, to stay positive. I had done everything that had been asked of me. I had kept up with my silent prayers with God. Even bargaining with him, as much as one can bargain with God. One is never quite sure he hears, and if he hears, will he listen?

Everything bad in my life had resolved itself with something good. I had been young when my daughter died. The pain of that was replaced by the joy of having two healthy sons. A bad marriage and a devastating divorce that left me penniless had been replaced with a successful career and a wonderful, loving relationship with Keith, my soul mate. Hadn't I been punished enough? I didn't deserve to be left at the end of my life as a disabled drug addict.

My thoughts were interrupted by Annie asking if she should set up the CPM machine. I shook my head no. Only the electromagnetic machine. I told her I just wanted to sleep. The machine was okay to use while I was napping. "When Keith comes up, tell him I said he should send you home and sign for your full hours. Oh, and pull the living room curtains closed." There was such sadness in Annie's eyes. This only added to the state I was in. I had to turn away.

I don't know how long I slept. What woke me was the urge to urinate, and possibly the sound of the television. Keith was sitting in a chair alongside the bed. I pointed to the commode but didn't speak.

"Can I get you something to eat? A cup of tea, perhaps?" he asked.

"Not hungry. But a cup of tea would be nice. And then get me my cell phone and charger. Don't say anything," I answered. He knew what I meant.

"What about the CPM machine?"

"Not tonight. One night without it won't matter," I answered with zero energy.

"I see you have the electromagnetic device on. Maybe it's time? You could take it off? You'll be more comfortable. I am sure you have already done ten hours."

"Okay," I agreed. "And my meds. You know I can't take them on an empty stomach."

"What about some toast?" he asked.

"Okay. But only one slice. When I've finished, I just want to sleep. Please leave the TV on."

My thoughts organized themselves. *Okay, if you are to be a cripple, you don't have to be a drug addict too. In any event, if you have to buy Oxy on the street, you'll go bankrupt.*

It's up to you, Elaine, I said to myself. *You and your brain.* I remember commending my brain. Without its assistance, I am not sure I could have had my leg make the progress it did. Well, the progress to move, not to heal. Could I change the message to send energy toward healing?

I made a decision to stop the Oxy. *I will put my self-created drug rehab program into effect tomorrow,* I promised. I had finally reached 88 degrees. Ninety was close. Instead of the oxycodone, I would take two extra-strength Tylenol with codeine (even though I was allergic to codeine). I would do it forty-five minutes before getting on the CPM machine. The pain didn't really start until I hit about 80 degrees. My idea was that I was strongest in the morning, and I would be better able to bear what I needed to endure.

The rest of the day, I slept the sleep of the dead. I don't even remember getting up to pee. Around 6:00 a.m., I heard Keith in the bathroom. And then I heard his footsteps down the hall. "Need some assistance to get to the potty?" he asked.

"Nope. Just need for you to stay nearby as always. When I am back on the bed, can you put up the kettle and make some tea?"

I knew Keith's tea would be strong. Keith always said Americans make tea that looks insipid. Brits make tea black, black tea that actually looks black. Then some cream to dilute it a little, and sugar, not artificial sweetener. I grew to like it that way. His mum always said, "Whatever ails you, a cup of tea will help."

"When Annie comes, why don't you go out? I know you have some things you need to do in the office," I suggested. "On the way home, could you please pick up some chocolate ice cream?" I added, with as charming a smile as I could muster. *See, my dear, I'm not depressed,* I was trying to show him. *I'll be okay. Today's a new day.*

I outlined my drug rehab plan to Annie. "I need to take two extra-strength Tylenol with codeine forty-five minutes before I go onto the CPM machine." I told her about my allergy and hoped aloud that I would not be so nauseous it would make me throw up. I asked her to bring me the Tylenol and a washcloth to bite down on as I didn't want to bite into my cheek. Joking, I added, "What I really need is a stick or piece of leather like in the old Westerns to position between my teeth. And John Wayne or Clint Eastwood to put it there would help!" I offered a weak smile as I took the tablets.

I started the CPM at 65, determined to keep raising the angle no matter what, until I could get to 90 degrees. Then I'd back down a bit and then ratchet it back up. I was determined not to give in to the pain, no matter how severe it got.

Annie was fully on board and supported my efforts.

"It's okay," she kept repeating. "Take my hand, squeeze it hard as you like. I've survived guys, big strong like oxen, who finally decided to face the devil, and watched as giant tears rolled down their faces. All you need is the will and you, sweets, will do it. Jesus will help you. Just keep prayin'."

"But I'm Jewish!" I pushed out between gritted teeth.

"Never you mind! So was he, until he converted!" And we both laughed.

This time Annie had to keep her eyes on the clock. Most of the time mine were pressed tightly closed and I was counting the seconds. It helped to be distracted. I did see the hand go around the face. I pushed to keep the CPM at 90 as much as I could, but by the end of the first hour, I was back down to 80.

At the end of the two-hour session, my palms were bleeding from the pressure of my nails digging into the skin and despite the washcloth, my cheeks were raw from gritting my teeth. But I had done it. My brain had cooperated. And my clock had assisted in measuring the degree of pain I could tolerate before having to lower the angle. Mission accomplished.

Annie applied a cold compress to my head and some antiseptic ointment with a topical pain killer to my hands and slipped two Oxys into my hand.

"Think of something pretty and look at the clock. See if you can wait one more hour to take them. Your decision, girl. Be strong. Maybe you can try to sleep? I know you are exhausted."

I knew I had to take the meds before the physical therapy session at the hospital because they would push me harder than I pushed myself. But I had broken the cycle and would do so again the next morning. Only Tylenol. No Oxy. Like the plan at Smokenders. Eliminate one and the rest will be easy.

Ultimately, I had Keith cancel the physical therapy appointment. I was in no mood, and I didn't know how much more pain I could endure that day.

When Keith came home and saw my hands, I explained to him what I'd done and why.

"I am so proud of you, babe," he said. Then he changed the topic. "It's Saturday. Do you want to go out? Over to the beach? Another cup of tea perhaps?"

"No. I need time to think and be quiet. And I need for you to forgive me. I know me better than anyone else, including you. I need the time to pass with no one or nothing, even you, to interrupt the process. Today will pass." Then, channeling my best Greta Garbo voice, I added "I *vant* to be alone!" and threw my hand across my forehead as I swooned back dramatically against the pillows.

I hoped with all my heart that Keith would understand. I asked for what I needed. "Just be here for potty and my meds on the written schedule."

Each day after that, I substituted the Tylenol for the Oxy in the morning and consciously lengthened the time in between other doses as well. Eventually, I was able to use Tylenol all the time (except for when I went to my physical therapy appointments). As I look back on it, I think trying to stop smoking was harder. It is possible that breaking the smoking addiction provided the pathway to breaking this one.

CHAPTER 23

GETTING PROACTIVE

The Sunday after I got the news that my bones weren't healing, Keith came into the living room, said good morning and that he would stand by while I went to the potty. With full-on optimism and energy in his tone, he slipped into his coaching voice and launched his plan.

"It is time to be proactive and not reactive! Your silent period is over. I'm going to make us a special breakfast. I am bringing you your iPad, and I want you to look up the best orthopedic surgeons in New York City. Make us a list of the best three. You'll call them Monday for an appointment.

"Then, you need to send a text and email to your friend Stanley and ask him to find out who his wife[3] would recommend as the best orthopedic surgeon there.

"After breakfast, I'll bring you the Tylenol and CPM machine. I know you're trying to eliminate your dependence on the Oxy. I'm not stupid. After living with you for all these years, I can read you

---

[3] A doctor at NYU medical center.

129

like a book. I'll get my ski mittens if you want to use them, which may protect your palms. I've made some extra ice packs." He smiled with that knowing look. Continuing, he said, "To change the subject, the weatherman says no humidity and warm temperatures will prevail today, so we're going to the beach around 4:00 p.m."

The word "prevail" stuck out of his soliloquy like a sore thumb. Not a word that any American would use. But Keith being Keith, sometimes his flowery use of language and his strong English accent still charmed me. To me, he was just Keith.

"The electromagnetic device is fully charged, so when you want it, just let me know," he continued. "And, one other thing, my darling. Now that your left leg is stronger, maybe we can see if you can get out of our bed onto the commode? I'm tired of sleeping alone and hate getting out of bed and going to the living room to watch you move from the bed to the commode. I know I am there as a safety. Your side of our bed is the one that will allow you to get left side out first. In the bedroom, if you can manage to get out of the bed, then at least I won't have that long walk down the hallway. And, as an added benefit, we'll be able to get rid of the hospital bed. What do you think of that?"

Wow. My man was impressive. He'd obviously been thinking about a lot of things while I was in retreat mode. I felt loved and cared for!

"Great plan for the day," I complimented him, pointing to the potty. "Sorry about yesterday. I just needed to get all that moping out of my system. I trained myself in the hospital that no matter what happened in the day, once those two hands of the clock were upon one another at midnight, when the second hand started to move to the right, I had a clean slate. No carryover. I watched those clock hands last night, love of my life; I need to tell you, I am over yesterday."

Our part of the beach was at the very end of Long Beach, going east. When we arrived late in the afternoon that Sunday, most families with small children had already departed, or were in the process of doing so. It was quiet. Calm. Peaceful.

The city had constructed mini boardwalks with benches at the end for people in wheelchairs, baby carriages, and beach buggies to get closer to the water. Keith sat on a bench and protectively turned me so that I was out of the way of anyone passing by. I wouldn't get bumped.

As I sat looking at the water, I saw a young woman, maybe in her twenties, coming toward me. She had the same brace as me, and her arm was in a cast. She used a crutch to help with walking. Alongside her was an older woman providing help, whom I assumed was her mother.

I watched this woman get off the sand and onto the boardwalk and said to her:

"Well, between the two of us, we have one good pair of legs!" We laughed together. "What happened to you?" I asked.

"Car accident." she said. "I was walking on Merrick Road and a car ran a light, hit me, and I was thrown 200 feet."

I gasped.

"Me too! Car accident! But I was in the car." I changed topics, "If you don't mind me asking, can you tell me your doctor's name and where he is located?"

"My first doctor was okay, but he had a terrible bedside manner. The doctor I am seeing now," she said as she gave me a huge smile, "is so handsome and so nice. Well, first thing I did was to look at his ring finger to see if he was married. He is. His name is Dr. Rozbruch, and he is chief of surgery at the Hospital for Special Surgery in Manhattan… Listen, I need to keep going. The beach is great, but it tires me out. Good luck!" She walked off with her mother.

"Good luck to you too," I said as I watched her go. I turned to Keith and said, "You are not going to believe this! That doctor is one of the three on my list!"

I remember that afternoon as clearly as I remember the day of the accident and the following day. We left the beach just as the sun was setting. A perfect New York summer sky. It was red and orange and then pink and purple. When the sun finally dipped to the horizon, the sky was ablaze in gold. The young woman and her information on Dr. Rozbruch, that blazing sunset, and the morning lecture from Keith were all signs that life could and would return to normal. Maybe soon?

CHAPTER 24

DOCTOR SEARCH

The phone was ringing just as we opened the door to our apartment. Keith ran for the phone.

"Stanley... for you...," he shouted. "He says he has some info for you from Marlene." I trusted Stanley's wife's judgement regarding referrals to any doctor affiliated with her at NYU Medical Center.

"Hi, my dear," Stanley greeted me in his traditional fashion. "Get yourself a pen and paper. Marlene says this guy has a great reputation." I scribbled while he listed off a name. "Call tomorrow, mention Marlene's name, and I am sure he will see you soon. Any problems with getting a quick appointment, and I'll have Marlene call him directly. In any event, how are you?"

"Fine," I answered. "Making progress."

"Great. I've got to go right now. I am at the marina and need to tidy up the boat. You know the drill. Call me and let me know how you make out. Oh, and tell Keith if he wants to crew next weekend, I can use an extra hand."

"Keith, Stan got me the name of another doctor at NYU Medical Center. I don't want to get my hopes up too high, but I have a really good feeling. I know you want to start dinner, but I'd like to get on the CPM machine. Can you set it up for me? And may I please have some water and the bottle with the Oxy?" I had only taken some extra-strength Tylenol so far during the day. "Oh, and my iPad, please."

"iPad?" he questioned.

"Yeah. I want to see if there is some info on what I should expect in the way of symptoms from breaking an addiction to Oxy. I am determined to cure myself. I don't think there's anything like Methadone to help. I think I will just have to tough it out."

The Oxycodone tablets my doctor prescribed were supposed to be taken every four to six hours. I knew I was addicted because I was taking them earlier and earlier and looked forward to getting them into my system, feeling that rush of relief. I was afraid that I wouldn't be able to stop taking them.

The first thing I read was that the symptoms of withdrawal would occur eight to twelve hours after the last dose. My plan was to gently wean myself off the drug like I had when I stopped smoking. If I could lengthen the time between doses, keep a schedule, and not take anything except Tylenol for the morning, I should succeed. I would use my clock to set alarms.

After dinner, Keith wheeled me into the bedroom. "Okay," he said, "here's the walker. Try the transfer to the bed. I think our bed is the same height as the bed in the physical therapy room at LBH. I'm right here. Close enough to catch you if you teeter a little. Take your time."

My left leg had gotten stronger. "Mission accomplished," I said as I lowered myself to the bed.

"Great, babe," Keith said, bubbling with excitement. "I'm getting the commode from the living room and will put it next to the bed. Look, see? I put lots of pillows to divide the bed between you and me so that I cannot hurt you in my sleep. At least I can hold your hand and bend over to kiss you good night."

I adored my husband and gave him a look to let him know that, as I teased, "Well, let's hope you don't snore too loudly and keep me awake!" And then I added, "And don't forget: you're still on potty duty, just without that long walk."

I should have slept really well seeing as I was back in my comfy bed, but I didn't. I needed to get accustomed to the feel of the bigger bed and the sounds of Keith's snoring and breathing. I kept waking up, looking at the clock, and hoping it would move faster so I could make those critical phone calls to set up appointments with the recommended orthopedists in the city. The idea of having a plan, being proactive, and actually doing something to help myself get back to normal, had activated adrenalin in my body. Endorphins were circulating. This was all good! Just made it harder to sleep!

At 9:30 a.m., I took the house phone and dialed the number for Dr. Rozbruch. I was both excited and nervous. Keith had taken this particular Tuesday morning off. Annie had bathed me, and I had put on a little makeup, even though no one could see me through the phone. It was a mental thing. Like looking your best when going for a job interview.

The phone rang several times. I was just starting to believe I'd dialed the wrong number when I heard a voice asking to where I wished to be directed. I asked for Dr. Rozbruch to make an appointment and was told he was at a different office, not in the hospital.

She transferred me and gave me the direct line info in case we were cut off.

After three rings, a pleasant voice answered. I had not asked the woman at the beach her name, so I simply told the receptionist that I was calling to make an appointment. The receptionist asked if I had ever been there before and then a series of questions regarding my condition. I learned that the person to whom I was speaking was named Rosa, and she told me it was my lucky day. She had a cancellation and asked if I could come the following Monday. I affirmed that I could indeed and began to buzz with excitement!

Rosa set me up for 10:00 a.m. and reminded me to bring ID, insurance card, and if it was from a car accident, the information on the insurance company. If I had been hospitalized, she wanted me to bring the papers from the hospital and the hospital information so she could get a release for my records. I asked for the address and some information about parking nearby before hanging up.

During this whole call, Keith was sitting right next to me and heard everything. He too thought it was lucky we could get in so quickly and suggested we test our luck by trying for an appointment with the second doctor on the same day. The two doctors were merely blocks away from each other on the upper east side of New York City. What luck! We got the appointment with the second doctor for the same afternoon. Clearly fate was with us!

Keith had to go to the office for the afternoon, but Annie was there to make me lunch and set up the CPM machine. I took the Tylenol and told Annie to make sure I had enough ice packs. I knew the ice would help dull the pain once the two hours on the CPM were completed.

Forty-five minutes later, I set the CPM to 80, and it wasn't long before I actually reached 90. The pain was less intense than the day before. I felt like the angels were smiling at me.

Dear God, I prayed. *Please don't let this be one of your jokes. Don't tease me. Haven't I suffered enough?* I prayed for courage and strength and that the week would pass quickly, and that there would be no other mishaps or hiccups. But that night, I learned God was not done with me yet.

CHAPTER 25

ZIG ZAGS IN MY EYES

JULY—4 MONTHS SINCE ACCIDENT

I don't remember what day of the week it was, just that it was night-time. I was on the phone with my long-time friend, Judy. I met Judy when I was sixteen years old. We caught up on all the small talk about families and were discussing my upcoming appointments in Manhattan. And then I was trying to explain to her the benefits of my new wheelchair cushion and I could not remember the word cushion. I could describe it, explain its function and all, but the word was not there. I wanted to tell her something specifically about the wheelchair and again, I could not remember what it was called. She asked me to put Keith on the phone.

After talking to Judy, Keith looked concerned said, "Judy told me you could not remember certain words and that your speech seemed slurred. She thinks you may be having a stroke. I'll get your sweatshirt; we're going over to the hospital. It's probably nothing, but we need to check it out." He was calm when he spoke to me and kept reassuring me and asking questions. Diagnosing and symptom-related questions.

"Do you feel numb anywhere?" he asked.

"No," I said, "but I do have a bad headache and I have those funny lightning things in both eyes. I can't see very well." At this point, I was really scared. Not at the panic stage yet. I told myself this was probably a reaction to the lessening of the Oxy in my system.

I started talking to my brain. Same as the other times I was facing something uncontrollable. *Okay, brain, whatever this is, you have to fix it.*

Long Beach Hospital is a small hospital. The ER wasn't busy. Once Keith told the nurse why we were there, she directed me into a bed in one of the emergency bays and immediately went to get the on-call doctor. The young doctor was efficient and worked to set up the machine to test for a stroke, as he listened to Keith explain the situation. When he finished, he said to me, "At this hour, we have no one here to interpret the results. Do not worry, the results have been sent to a central service to be read, and we should have them in about forty-five minutes. I want you to raise your arms, one at a time, and now touch your nose with both hands. Do you feel numb anywhere? Tingles?"

"No," I replied as I followed all his instructions. "Doctor, I have a splitting headache. Can I have some Tylenol?"

"When did you get the headache?"

"Maybe an hour ago. Sometimes I get ocular migraines. You know, little zig zags in front of my eyes. Sometimes the zig zags go away. Sometimes I get this terrible headache. I got the zig zags when I was on the phone with my friend."

"I'm glad you told me that. We need to see the test results before I can give you anything, but I'll have the nurse get you an ice pack. Sometimes that helps the headache. We will continue to monitor you and if you feel anything out of the ordinary, you need to let me know right away."

I was hooked up to the usual machines, and my blood pressure and heart rate were beeping across the screens as I tried to avoid looking as panicked as I felt. I didn't want to let on to Keith how scared I was. All the anxiety temporarily made me forget about any other pains.

I closed my eyes and drifted back to the time that Keith had gone to Florida to open our second office. Back then, we couldn't afford the fare to visit each other regularly, so we hardly saw one another. That was when I started getting these massive headaches. Along with the headaches came rolling blackouts in my memory. I always prided myself on my memory. I hardly ever wrote anything down. I could be legless and armless, but never mindless. At that time, I told myself, if I had a mental illness, I would bow out.

My internist had sent me to a neurologist, who could not find anything clinically wrong with me. He asked me what was different in my life, and I told him about Keith being away. He said that I was experiencing the same symptoms one sometimes faces with the death of someone really close. Other symptoms were loss of memory, disorientation, changes in sleep pattern, even loss of appetite. He gave me a prescription for my headache and told me to follow the same routines and patterns daily. Put your keys and glasses in the same place consistently. Carry a notebook and keep notes about what you should be doing and when. He said the headaches would subside and the memory would get better. He was right.

The ice from the ER doc helped a bit. A nurse came in several times to check me and the monitors. When the doctor finally appeared again, I learned that the tests didn't show anything. He surmised that my disorientation could have been the result of a migraine, which sometimes has that effect, and wanted me to see a neurologist. After promising to call the neurologist himself and get me in to see her immediately, he told me to go home, rest, and that he would follow up with me the next day to see how I felt. Tearing off a page from his prescription pad with the name, address, and phone number of the neurologist, the doctor said I should call and set up the appointment for the following day and to make sure they send him the results.

"Thank God," I said, turning to Keith.

I thanked the doctor and asked, "Hey, doc, what about the Tylenol for my headache? Can I have that now?"

"Yes," he said, smiling. "Go home, get into bed, try to sleep. That will help the headache. Keep up with the ice too. Still got lightning flashes?"

"No, just a really bad headache."

I wondered if the stress of my pending appointments in the city was causing the same kind of zig zag eyes and headaches I had started to get when Keith was away from me, or if all of this was a reaction to my withdrawal from the Oxycodone. I just prayed that it would all go away by morning.

In the car going home, I thought about the saying about whatever doesn't kill you makes you stronger. My immediate reaction was BULLSHIT! My body hurt all over. Not just my head. Sometimes I was up, but mostly, lately, I was down. It was all getting to be too much. There were too many things happening that created negative thoughts, like maybe it would have been better if I had died. All of this would be over.

But then I thought about Keith. Would he have been able to survive the guilt if I had actually died? I didn't think so. Was that why I survived?

It seemed like everything was getting more and more difficult, and the current trip to the emergency room just reinforced that idea. What if I never walked again? My hopes were hinging on those two doctors in the city and what they would tell me. But what if? I interrupted my own downward spiral and thought, *I can't think about this now.*

Once we were home, I had Keith call Judy to give her the update. "Tell her I am okay, and that I am resting and will call her tomorrow," I instructed him.

The next day I met with the neurologist recommended by the ER doctor. My visit with Dr. Gray included a session of being wired up with electrodes so that I looked like the Bride of Frankenstein. I still have the picture Keith took of me.

Dr. Gray said that I had some white spots on my brain, but no more than normal for a woman of seventy years. Clinically she couldn't find anything wrong.

"But I definitely think you are suffering from PTSD," she added. "And some of the symptoms you just experienced may be directly related to your accident. Although, I do think this was an ocular migraine. Disorientation is a common experience.

"If you had not been on the phone, you would not have known any of this. So, in a way, it was a good thing. Now you know your brain appears to be normal. Your records show you have gone through a very traumatic experience, a major car accident and substantial hospital time. And your husband has told me of the fears and symptoms you have every time you need to get into a car. Deep intakes of breath, sometimes losing your breath entirely, sometimes hands shaking.

"I suggest it would be in your best interest to see a psychologist. I can recommend someone who is excellent, right here in Long Beach. His name is Dr. Temple, and he is located on Park Avenue."

"Okay," Keith said. "I will make sure Elaine gets the appointment. PTSD is something I never thought about. Everyone, including me, just raves over how well she seems to have handled all of this. I know my wife. She is the strongest person I know. I know both of us are relieved nothing is wrong with her brain. The trauma hospital never tested anything regarding her head, as far as I know." Keith looked at me, and I nodded in agreement.

I made an appointment with Dr. Temple, who had availability that Friday afternoon.

CHAPTER 26

THE FEARS THAT PLAGUE US

For the rest of the week, my spirits began to lift. There were many changes happening around me. The hospital bed was removed from the living room, and my home returned to looking like my home again. Davie, one of the physical therapists, measured my knee bend and told me that not only had I reached 90, I had extended to 92! That was really good news.

The therapist said that since I was at a consistent 90 degrees, I didn't need the CPM machine any longer! That was even better news.

At this point, I only needed the Oxy for the physical therapy sessions. If I cut out one entire dose and took only extra-strength Tylenol in between, maybe I could use my brain again to concentrate on pushing the pain outside of my body. Mind over matter. If I made my leg move with my mind, could I do the same with kicking a drug habit? Maybe. Just maybe I could.

That good news came right before Davie started me on some more intense training! You could see I was "riding" that high when Davie put me up on a bicycle and wanted to see how I would do with the pedals. Getting up onto the bike was the most difficult part, as no weight could be put on my right leg. It took two therapists to get me up and into the seat. Try as I might, I could not make any rotation going forward using only my left leg. Only backwards. My right leg just went along for the ride, resting on the pedal. Both therapists said in unison, "Don't worry, you will eventually do it."

How many times had I heard that before? And, yet, they were right. I eventually could do everything the therapists and doctors had told me I would be able to. Lessons learned: Don't doubt yourself. Have faith. The whole concept of a positive attitude was in my nature, so instead of dwelling on what I couldn't do, I challenged myself to accomplish all that I could.

After the physical therapy session, Keith announced that he too had some news that would make me happy.

"From now on, I am going to take every Wednesday off as well as every Friday. We'll need to tell Annie that she'll only be needed three days a week. And, of course, we won't need her this Monday, your big day with the doctors."

I was determined to use only Tylenol and only just before the therapy sessions. I continued applying ice. But now, without the Oxy, I could use the ice in another, more pleasurable way. I could use it to chill my wine or vodka. Oh, how I missed being able to have a drink once in a while!

My increased arm and left leg strength gave me the ability to not spend so much time sitting. Annie or Keith was always with me to

146

make sure I didn't have another near miss with touching down my right foot. I would hop around on my one healed foot, using my arms to propel the walker forward. Walkers at the time did not have the seats or baskets that they do now.

However, necessity being the mother of invention, my bra strap became a good place to hold my phone (in addition to holding up my boobs). I never had to wonder where I left the phone—it stayed close to my heart, and I didn't have to worry about someone walking away with it without me knowing!

A small canvas bag hung like a feedbag around my neck. This enabled me to carry my makeup, glasses, and anything else lightweight. I still hadn't figured out how to carry a drink around with me, but you can only do so much!

Even though I was now sleeping in my own bed, sleep was still not coming easily. At times it truly was Keith's snoring, but it was mostly that my mind became more active in the quiet time. That's when all of the fears of remaining immobile would manifest themselves. Part of me was excited to see the doctors on Monday, and part was filled with dread. What if there was no hope of recovery? What would I do? And how would that impact my relationship with Keith? Would he get tired of caring for me and caring about me? That scared me more than anything.

Keith was still the same Keith, or so it seemed. I could not read his mind. He was not cross with me, ever. I had no reason to think what I had been thinking, no reason to doubt him, but well... we had been together for ten years and married for almost eight of them. I never expected to be married again after my divorce. It just happened. Ever since the beginning, Keith had always put me before anything and anyone else. We became an "us" in every sense of the word. I was a whole person with him, not a dependent.

The fear that he would leave me became intertwined with the fear of never walking again.

And so, it was my fears that were primarily on my mind, and not the PTSD, when at 2:00 p.m. that Friday, Keith and I entered Dr. Temple's office for my psychology appointment.

Our session with Dr. Temple was mostly spent catching him up to speed on all that had transpired and the issues I was having that the neurologist felt were accident- and PTSD-related. I shared the fears I had when I got in a car, and he taught me some relaxation exercises to do as part of my daily routine, but also some specifically to be used in anxiety-producing situations.

CHAPTER 27

DR. BLUE EYES

84 DAYS SINCE THE ACCIDENT

Sunday, I overheard Keith on the phone with Mitch.

"Just a heads-up and a reminder, I'm taking your mom to the city tomorrow. She'll be seeing two orthopedic surgeons, and I just hope that one of them will be able to help her. She doesn't say much, but I know it's starting to really get to her. In error, she sent me a mass email she has sent to the staff requesting them to keep her in their prayers this weekend. This is definitely not like your mom. Give her a call later. And if you could, do me a favor and call David and let him know about tomorrow? Send my best to Kim, and if you speak to the kids, tell them to keep writing to Elaine. Their postcards and letters from camp lift her spirits."

Monday morning, I was up before the 6:00 a.m. beep of the alarm. Three alarms were set. One on each iPhone and one on the clock.

I had decided to wear a dress (which was more like a long tee shirt) so that I would only have to lift it for any x-rays or the exam.

We knew that the regular Monday traffic into Manhattan would be augmented by the summertime people returning to work early Monday morning from the beach towns at the east end of Long Island.

Before we headed to the city, before the car even started, I needed to run through the relaxation technique the therapist taught me. All that added to the time we needed to allow for travel was stressing me out.

"Don't give me a large cup of coffee," I shouted to Keith, who was in the kitchen. "The less fluid I have in my system, the better." The maximum duration I could control my bladder was about four hours. I elected to put on a Depends just in case.

Once in the car, Keith said, "Okay, just let me know when we can get going. Is it okay for me to put on 1010 WINS in the car so I can keep abreast of the traffic?"

"Of course, silly," I said. "Just get me to the church on time."

"Church?"

"Yeah. Remember that scene from *My Fair Lady*? Or was it some other show?"

"Okay, my dear," he said. "Whatever you say. That can be researched later. Your chauffeur is ready, willing, and able. Off we go."

The trip had several nasty short stops, but the breathing technique Dr. Temple had shown me helped keep me relatively calm, with fewer of the deep gasps that vexed Keith.

The parking garage was only a few doors down from the office of Dr. Rozbruch. The parking attendant directed us off to the side of the ramp that lead into the garage, so Keith could get me into the wheelchair and positioned under the protective overhang of the building. When he came out of the garage about ten minutes later and we started up the street, I expressed my need for a bathroom. After about two and a half hours on the road, plus the waiting time for Keith to park the car and my preparatory relax time, well, my bladder was nearing its limit.

Just as we turned off the elevator on the second floor, there was a sign indicating the restroom. "I'm desperate to go," I told Keith. Keith said not to worry, that he was there to help.

So, here I was in the most prestigious orthopedic hospital in the world, and I found myself wanting to shoot the plumber. The toilet itself was very low. The unisex handicapped accessible bathroom was a large, very well-lit space, with one toilet and a sink. However, the only grab bar was attached to the tile on the wall opposite my right hand. In order for me to be able to sit, I had to stand up out of the wheelchair, facing the toilet, holding onto Keith's arms; then pivot so I was facing the opposite direction, never letting go of Keith; hike my dress up and pull my undies down—all with my left hand; and, using the strength I had in my left leg, bend my knee in order to have Keith ease me down onto the seat. Gravity was a big help there.

But getting up and back into the wheelchair? THAT was a whole other story. While I held onto the grab bar with my left hand, Keith faced me, put his arms under my arms, locked his hands behind my back, and literally had to pull me up to standing, while I used all of the strength in my left leg to get upright. I was terrified I would fall or twist in a way that would have sent my right foot on to the floor or dropped me back onto the toilet. If there had been another grab bar—

maybe an upside down, U-shaped pipe (bicycle rack style) alongside the toilet in addition to the grab bar attached to the wall—I wouldn't have been so terrified, and my left leg wouldn't have had to work so hard. My arms would have taken some of the weight burden.

"Well," I said once back into the wheelchair, "now I know what God had planned for me." Keith looked at me quizzically. "I am to be the best designer of toilets for handicapped people in the world! We will make a fortune," I said, smiling. "It's either that, or God has to give women an alternate plumbing system." That remark sent him into fits of laughter, which broke the tension that had built up in trying to do a "simple" void.

Keith pushed me down the hall but once at check-in, the receptionist advised us that we needed to go *back* down the hallway, turn right, and enter a room marked "x-rays."

Just thinking about those x-rays, even now, makes me shudder with fear. I was given a walker and positioned myself, at the technician's request, to stand in front of a screen. He instructed me to place my damaged leg on the floor with no weight on it, then pivot around on it, but he said I could not hold on to the walker while the x-ray was being taken.

"No, no," I cried. "If any weight goes onto that right leg, it could shatter more, and then I'll have no hope of being anything but a cripple for the rest of my life."

"Okay," he said, "I'll help you to get into position with your back against the wall, and I'll help you to get your right foot into position so I can take the picture. It is only fifteen seconds out of your life. Practice just easing it on the floor."

"It hasn't touched the floor in months," I said, half crying, my voice quavering.

"Listen," he said. "You are strong, and you can hold onto the wall for balance, but it must be on the floor. Now take a deep breath and remember, you cannot move."

I did it and then my left leg went into spasms. When it calmed down, he helped me to turn sideways.

"Can't we do this where I can lay down?" I begged.

"These are Dr. Rozbruch's orders. Put your right hand up on the wall. Now let go of the walker and take a deep breath." As soon as I heard the click, he was there in a matter of seconds. Holding me up, he dragged me over to the x-ray table, brought me my wheelchair and a glass of water.

"Well, Miss Champion," he said as he pushed me out of the room, "you get my Monday gold star."

Keith took one look at me and asked what happened.

"You're white as a ghost!" he observed. All I could do was to motion with my hand as if to say "not now."

As we entered the waiting room, a young woman asked if I was Miss Rosendorf, and once confirmed, she took us to an examination room where she assured me I would be more comfortable. She then inquired; would we like coffee, juice, water? I asked for juice and Keith requested coffee.

Within a short time, a tall man with a white lab coat entered the room and introduced himself. "I'm Dr. Quig, assistant to Dr. Rozbruch. While we wait for the x-rays and for Dr. Rozbruch to come in, I will ask you some questions. I see you've brought your films and reports, but as you now know, we take our own x-rays here."

There were the usual questions: What medications are you on? Describe your pain. What do you take for it? Etc. The question session lasted about forty minutes.

When the door opened again, a very handsome, youthful-looking man (fully living up to the hype of my boardwalk beach friend), said, "I am Dr. S. Robert Rozbruch, and I am glad to meet you." I instantly knew why the young woman from the beach was so taken with him. He was very soft-spoken and had the kindest blue eyes, with dimples in each cheek.

He told us he had been with the Hospital for Special Surgery (HSS) for ten years (a position offered to him after his internship) and he was currently Chief of Surgery. My instincts told me I was in the right place with the right doctor, but I knew I would still keep the appointment with the other doctor in the afternoon.

He looked at Keith and said, "I assume you are the husband?"

"Yes?"

"You have a very attractive wife."

"I know," Keith replied. "I am a lucky man. She is the love of my life, and I hope you can help her."

"I want to show you your x-rays," he said, turning and sitting down in a chair. "I am sorry for any discomfort, physical or mental, but I have my reason for making you stand up for the films."

And there it was, my right leg, in "living color." I could see the holes in the bone. I could see the plate and some of the screws. And I could see the small amount of tissue surrounding the bone. My leg had shrunk down to nothing. I was horrified, sad, frightened.

"The damage is extensive. I want to see you stand up like you did in the x-ray room, and place that right leg on the floor. But first, I'm going to remove the brace. You can hold onto the examination table for support. Now hold on, I need for you to turn completely around. Pivot on your left foot," he instructed.

I moved, ever so slowly and with great caution.

"I see you have a large scar on that left ankle. What happened?"

"I had a broken ankle from the accident. I don't know how it got broken, but I know it was pinned under the dashboard. The doctors at the hospital told me it was a bad break but a clean one."

"How long was the cast on?"

"About four to five weeks, I think."

"And is it now totally healed?"

"Yes, but still fairly weak, although now I have some muscle back."

"Okay, let me help you to sit back down," he said. He looked first at me, and then at Keith, and then back at me.

"Let me tell you what my specialty is: It is bone lengthening. But I also do other kinds of surgery, such as bone grafts, which you may have read about. An analysis of the x-rays and the fact that there appears to be no healing is of great concern to me, especially considering your age. You don't look seventy," he assured me, smiling.

"Good genes, I guess. But there are many days I feel seventy—maybe more. I don't think I can adjust to not being able to resume my old life. Or at least, at a minimum not being able to walk. I was so sure, after my ankle healed so quickly, that my leg would do the same."

He took my hand, perhaps to comfort me. I think I was more surprised than anyone now that I had verbalized my fears. I hadn't ever done that with Keith, or Dr. Temple, or even with myself. *How strange*, I thought.

"I would like to try a bone graft and see what happens." He saw I was about to ask him something, but he just continued. "We can do this one of two ways; I can use the bones of a cadaver that have been irradiated. Or I can remove some of the bone from your pelvic girdle. The first way, there is less chance of infection, but more chance of rejection, since the bone is not from your body. The opposite is true if I use your bone. In addition, I will add antibiotics and some artificial bone and then we will see. Until I am able to operate, I cannot know exactly what I will find."

"Why has the bone remained in the same state for so many months?" I asked, almost afraid to hear the answer.

"There could be a low-grade infection not evidenced in your blood work, or the capillaries may be so badly broken that they cannot assist in getting the blood into the bone, or it could be your age, or a combination of the three." It seemed to me I'd heard these same thoughts from my other doctors.

"Because of the length of time that there has been no growth of bone, I would want to do this as soon as possible. And if that doesn't work, well, we can see what else can be done to get that bone to heal, or start to grow, so the holes can fill in. See Rosa, my scheduler, on the way out and get her to give you a date. Tell her 'first available.' Ask her for my email address, and any questions you have, send me an email." As he rose to go, he turned, bent down, and gave me a gentle hug. He whispered in my ear, "In this hospital, failure is not an option."

Keith wheeled me down to Rosa's desk. She looked on the computer to find the first date available, and it wasn't until the end of September.

"That's kind of far into the future. Dr. Rozbruch said he wanted to operate on Elaine as soon as possible," Keith persisted. "Are you sure there is nothing available before then? That's two months away." She seemed at a loss.

Keith suddenly rose up and headed down the hall to chase down Dr. Quig. I could not hear what was being said, but it looked like Keith had turned on his best salesman charm and was working his magic. It looked as if he may have succeeded because when he reached Rosa's desk again, he said, "Go ahead and put us in for the date you have open, but Dr. Quig told me to call here around 2:00 p.m. today and if he is not available to ask for you. Can you give me your extension?"

As we left, he bent down and whispered in my ear, "I think we will get an earlier date. Cross your fingers."

One more trip to the restroom was required before Keith pushed me the five blocks to our next appointment at the second surgeon's office. We determined that walking would be faster than hailing a cab, moving me from wheelchair to cab seat, folding the wheel-chair and storing it in the trunk, dealing with New York City traffic snarls, and then doing it in reverse on the other end. It was a sunny day, not too warm, so I rather enjoyed the walk. Of course, Keith was pushing me, so I got to enjoy the scenery without working too hard.

Keith signed me in and held my file at the ready to give to Sara, the doctor's assistant, when she called us in.

Some forty-five minutes later, Sara appeared and took us into a small office where she asked many of the same questions I had answered just hours before. She then escorted us back to the waiting room and said the doctor would see us shortly.

We waited and waited and waited. I was getting upset, and then angry. Maybe we should just leave? Keith didn't want to leave.

"What if this doctor tells you the same thing and can operate sooner? You know he came highly recommended," he said.

Two o'clock arrived and Keith went to call Dr. Quig. Rosa told him Dr. Quig would call him back in an hour.

I was again nearing the limit of my bathroom time, when Sara finally came to escort us to an examination room. When the NYU

Medical Center doctor walked in, he was older than Dr. Rozbach and much more businesslike.

"I have reviewed your file and all of the x-rays and I see that your injuries, although quite extensive, may respond to a bone graft." He went on to explain the procedure, all the pros and cons of using irradiated bone from a cadaver vs. using my own.

"Normally, I would not be discussing any dates with you, but the conference I was to attend in about three weeks' time has just been cancelled. Sara will be in to explain the pre-op, when and where it should be done, and you can discuss the dates with her. Do you have any questions for me?"

"Yes. Which of the two ways you discussed do you feel would be the most beneficial?"

"My recommendation would be for you to use your own, even though this would be two independent operations done at the same time. There would be less chance of rejection, and hopefully a greater chance of success. Talk it over with your husband and advise Sara of your decision." At that, he just got up and left the room.

There was such a huge difference between the two appointments and the doctors. I said a silent prayer, asking God to intervene. I really wanted Dr. Rozbruch to do the surgery, but also thought that the longer I waited... well...

On the way to ladies' room, I was literally about to burst, when Keith's phone rang. It was Dr. Quig. As I was doing my business, I heard Keith say, "I should speak to Rosa and get all the info for August 8th? The operation will be on August 8th at 8 o'clock in the morning.... Yes, we're still in the city and parked near your office.... Okay, I'll see Rosa and pick up the paperwork. Thank you. Thank you! You have just made my day. And Elaine's!"

Keith turned to me with so much excitement in his voice and face.

"How do you feel?"

"Relieved, in more ways than one!" I joked with him.

"Let's get you something quick to eat," Keith said once we were outside. He rattled off his plan for the rest of the day. "Hopefully, we can still beat the rush hour traffic. I noticed a small café on the way over here, which would be perfect. I'll run up and get the paperwork from Rosa, and then we can start home. Babe, you look exhausted. I know this day has been very trying and stressful for both of us. I'm sorry the only thing I could do to help was hold your hand. I love you, you know. More than anyone or anything and I am sorry," Keith said.

"For what?" I asked, perplexed.

"For putting you in this position. I was the one driving. Remember?"

When I looked up at him, he was wiping his eyes. I stayed silent. I could not deny what he said was true. The love part, the blame part, and his remorse. He had finally voiced what I knew he was feeling. This was a big day for us on so many levels.

Monday ended much the way it began. Keith called Mitch. Mitch's reaction was to ask if we needed anything. I explained what I had to do for pre-op back at the hospital and that I needed to call for those appointments now that I had a surgical date.

"How do you feel?" Mitch asked me. A mother knows her children best, and I could tell by his tone that the question was loaded with more than just the simplicity of the words.

"Listen," I said. "I am feeling many things. Anticipation and hopeful that the bone graft will take and a bit apprehensive about the operation. Well two operations really, as I had explained to you. I am fully aware of the risks. The worry is that the desired results will not be achieved, and I will need... well, let's not talk about that. I need to stay positive. Anyway, I need to phone your brother.

159

The day has been a bit much, and I am tired. I'll keep you informed. Not to worry."

"Mom." Mitch didn't hang up. "Do you need for me to be at the hospital?"

"No. Your office is only a cab ride away, and Keith will be there. He'll keep you informed. I love you." He responded the same, and we hung up.

The call to David was a little longer. Unlike his brother, who is a man of few words, David required all of the details.

"I'm coming up, Mom."

I told him there was no need to do that, but he insisted that he could work out of the New York office.

"That's not necessary," I insisted. "Stay in Miami. Didn't you tell me that the partners from our office in Peru were planning to visit in August? If you are here, I will only have to worry about you. And you cannot cancel any appointment with the partners. It will not sit well. Keith will keep you informed."

"Okay, Mom; have it your way. You usually do." And we both laughed. David continued, "So, how will you spend the next few weeks?"

"I don't think I need to go to physical therapy. I'll check. Watch for a text from the surgeon with details and hospital information." And then I launched into the reason our calls always took longer—the business information my son needed to know. I wanted him to keep the Miami staff up to speed on my status, finish the London deal once I'd concluded all the legal contract stuff, have him take over supporting the NY staff that I managed remotely, and so on. Yes, even with all the physical therapy and CPM machine and electromagnetic machine, while my body was working, my mind was busy managing business affairs from home.

I concluded with "Need to get some rest. Kiss and hug my grand-daughter for me. Tell her I love and miss her. Love you too." And then I hung up and shut my eyes for a while.

On Tuesday, I called the HSS for the pre-op appointment. The paperwork stated that for patients and family, special arrangements could be made at the New York Presbyterian Guest Facility at the Helmsley Medical Tower, which was next door to the hospital. I booked a room for August 7th through 10th. The rooms were set up with a fully equipped kitchen, coffee makers, and daily housekeeping services. To get to the hospital itself, one only needed to go out the side building door, cross the street, and locate the entry door to into the hospital.

Wednesday afternoon, when Keith handed me the mail, there was an extraordinary and unexpected two-page handwritten letter from Dr. Rozbruch. He said I was the most delightful seventy-year-old he had every met and stated that he admired my courage and attitude. He would see me on the 8th. When I showed the letter to Keith, he laughed.

"The doctor said you are delightful? Well, that's a new adjective for you. Most adjectives are usually attributed to your nickname 'Dragon Lady.' Only kidding, only kidding."

I had spent a great deal of the previous thirty years in the East Asia and Southeast Asia. Several of my business partners gave me that name. I don't remember who said it first. It was not to describe the characteristics of the Dragon Lady in the Dick Tracy comics (although sometimes it was). I was a female who had been success-ful in a man's world. The transportation industry is male-dominated. I needed to be strong and demanding of the agents in order to bring success to them. The name Dragon Lady from them was a measure of respect. In the Chinese zodiac, Dragons are the strongest sign and symbolize character traits such as ambition and authority. Dragons live by their own rules, which usually produces success. I think that was a fair assessment of me.

Keith continued reading and concluded that since the note was handwritten, it was personal; no intermediary secretary involved. Whatever the doctor wrote was from the heart. Keith thought it was probably unique that the doctor wrote such a personal note.

"A credit to you, my darling. Especially for someone you have only met for the first time. But, just remember, you (and he) are already married. So please—" He winked. "—I won't take kindly to you two fooling around." I felt heat rise in my cheeks.

Years later, after Keith had passed away, there came another handwritten letter. I had made a donation in Dr. Rozbruch's name for research. I sent the doctor information about the donation, along with a letter advising him about my plans to write this book about my experiences. He thanked me and assured me that the money would be used for research. The last sentence of that letter read, "I am glad to hear you are well. Knowing you and Keith has enriched my life. Take care." I held onto this letter and put away safely. I hope one day I can find that first letter.

CHAPTER 28

I Finally Admit
the Truth

Friday, a little before 2:00 p.m., Keith brought me for my second visit to Dr. Temple. Dr. Temple greeted both of us and asked Keith about how things were going with the car rides. Keith said they were a bit better. Dr. Temple asked Keith to come back in an hour. The doctor wanted a private session with me. He told Keith, "From now on it will be just the two of us unless I feel there is a reason to include you back into the sessions."

As the door closed, the doctor asked what was new? How I was feeling? Was I doing the breathing exercises? Were they helping? And so on. He suggested that I use the same breathing exercises I used for the car rides anytime I was under stress. I told him about my next fear.

"I am scheduled for a bone graft on August 8th. I'm a bit scared. I received no promises, but I feel like it will be successful."

"Why is that?

"It's the date." He looked puzzled. "The date is 8/8 and the operation is scheduled for 8 a.m. Three eights." That didn't seem to clarify anything for him, so I continued, "In my business, I spent a lot of time in the Far East, especially in China and Hong Kong. The Chinese believe that two and eight are lucky numbers. And now I have three of them. Three eights, I mean."

"I wish you the best of luck. We only have a few more sessions before your operation. Today I want to concentrate on you, and maybe find out about some of your repressed fears and other things that may evidence themselves.

"In the last session, I could see the love and respect you and Keith have for one another. Do you feel that there is any change in your relationship?"

"Change?" I asked. "In what way?"

"Attitudes mainly."

"I need to think about that," I responded.

He waited a few minutes and when I did not continue, he looked at me and said, "Elaine, I am going to be very blunt. Do you blame Keith for what happened? For the fact that your life is so different and for the fact that after so many months, you are still unable to walk?"

I could feel the heat of tears on my face. I still didn't answer. Dr. Temple pushed a glass of water towards me. He urged me to drink some water and take my time before answering.

"Yes," I finally blurted out. "I know it was an accident, but he was driving, and the day was clear, but sometimes when he drives..."

"Yes. What about sometimes when he is driving?"

"I don't want to talk about it."

"You need to face this and not feel guilty about your thoughts. It is normal."

"Yes, I know it was an accident."

164

"It's not only fear of another accident or the memory of the accident that did happen, but the guilt you feel because deep down; you do blame him and you don't want to face it. And that's the reason for the gasping and intake of air when Keith is driving. Somewhere in your subconscious, you're hoping the sounds will make him stop driving. Your body is responding to those messages from your brain. Does that make any sense to you?" he asked.

I nodded, yes.

"Facing your true feelings, coming to grips with that, is what we need to work on together. You've suppressed them because you can never verbalize them for fear it will destroy your relationship. You're now dependent on him for so many more things than ever before, and this dependence is adding to the problem of suppression.

"Now that you've finally admitted this to yourself and to me, we can move forward with a plan. Perhaps you can arrange for someone else to drive you wherever you need to go?" Dr. Temple paused for a moment, before adding, "Just sit a few minutes calmly and do your breathing, and then we can continue."

CHAPTER 29

PRE-SURGERY

106 DAYS SINCE THE ACCIDENT

The night before my operation, Keith made a reservation at a small Italian bistro down the street from the hotel and hospital. It was a lovely family-style restaurant, small but not crowded. They were able to seat us so my wheelchair would not get bumped by passersby and waiters.

Keith and I spoke about things in general, both of us trying to pretend this was a normal date night like we used to have. Finally, Keith went there.

"Well, how do you feel?" he asked. "Are you nervous?"

"Of course, I'm nervous. But only a little. Apprehensive would better describe how I feel. And hopeful that it will work. You know, I don't remember anything about the surgeries I had in the trauma hospital. I haven't got a clue what an actual operating room looks like. Well, of course, there are the ones on the medical television shows, but maybe they don't really look like that at all.

"Just to put your mind at ease, for now, I'm trying to not think about it at all. I don't think this will be the case in the morning. And remember: we need to be there at six, so best we set the alarms to wake us at about five. Now, honey, how about another drink? I believe they will be putting me on an antibiotic, so my drinking will be nonexistent when I get home. At least for a while."

As my darling motioned to the waiter for more drinks, and he took my hand in his and said, "You know I love you more than anything. More than all the tea in China. More than all the stars in the sky. More than life itself. And, as much as sometimes you act like my mother, boss lady—" He smiled. "—I truthfully don't know what I would do without you." That just about said it all, and I felt so lucky to have this wonderful man in my life.

We tucked into bed at about midnight, after setting the phones and my little alarm clock to wake us. Doubling down, we left a wake-up call with the hotel as well.

Our sleeping positions had been altered, due to the brace on my leg. Keith's arm was always under my pillow and the other around my shoulder or touching my arm. We had gotten used to putting some pillows over the brace to prevent any further injury to my leg. And both of us would fall asleep on our left sides. Especially that night, it was a comfort to feel him spooning me and to listen to his breathing. He fell asleep rather quickly.

I did not fall asleep so readily. Somewhere in the back of my mind, all of my jumbled thoughts fell over each other trying to come together. I was not afraid of death. My fear, or should I say my concern, was for Keith. We had never discussed *what if*. I knew in my heart that, whenever one of us would depart from this earth, it should not be me first. I knew I had the strength to overcome, but I felt in my heart that he would be devastated and would not handle it well at all.

I decided to talk to God, in my mind, not aloud. I asked for the strength to get through the operation in the morning. If it was not his plan that I should walk again, I would accept it. If that was the case, I needed guidance on how to overcome that challenge and how to reorder my life. But mostly, I asked God not to let me die, because I knew Keith was not ready to be without me. That was the last thought I had before the alarms started going off, so somehow, I had managed to get some sleep after all.

The sun was not quite up yet when we exited the hotel and crossed the street to the hospital. We proceeded without talking, up to the floor where I needed to check in. There were many forms to sign, photos made of the insurance cards, a copy taken of my living will and power of attorney naming Keith, and finally, the form that confirmed I would pay the fee for the private room (to which the clerk attached a copy of my credit card). We were advised that in a very short time, we would be escorted into a large room and put in an assigned cubicle, where several doctors would come to see me, as well as the anesthesiologist.

I said to Keith as we waited, "I hope the private room is one that overlooks the river and the FDR. We can wave to one another on your way back into the city from the office at JFK.

"Once the operation is over, a few hours away from here will do you good. Jill should be here soon. I enlisted her to hold your hand. Joke. Joke," I told him, laughing. Jill is one of my closest friends, and I had asked her to make sure Keith was okay. I didn't know what was going to happen during surgery. I was seventy years old going under the knife, and wanted to be sure he had someone with him, just in case.

When Jill arrived, I handed her some envelopes with notes I had written to be distributed upon my death. I didn't want to leave words unsaid. It gave me some sense of security and completion to leave my thoughts for each important person in my life.

To Keith, I wrote: "Do not blame yourself for this. Should the end result be not what is desired, take care of yourself and stay close to the children. It has certainly been some trip. More than I could ever have hoped for or imagined. I will love you forever." It was simply signed, Me.

The nurses interrupted our silent reveries with bustling activities and preparations. I had to be changed into a gown. Head and foot coverings were added like the final jewelry accessories when you're heading out to a ball, the last step after your dress is zippered closed. The anesthesiologist visited and explained everything that would happen in the operating room. And then it was time to go.

Kisses, a big hug, and "See you soon, darling. Best of luck," wishes from Keith.

I handed Keith my thin, yellow gold 10th anniversary wedding band. "Put this around your neck so you don't lose it."

As the nurse wheeled me on a gurney down the hall and through double doors into another hallway, I did breathing exercises to calm myself.

When the double doors whooshed open in front of us and we entered the surgical theater, I saw the huge clock with my friends— the minute and hour hands. I sighed with relief. My clock. My anchor. I would be okay. I knew all would go fine, and that death was not coming for me on this particular day. I knew that God had more things in store for me and wasn't done with me yet.

CHAPTER 30

SURGERY

Looking around the operating room, I could see that the television medical dramas were mainly accurate in their depictions. There were three large lights hung from the ceiling. A bank of monitors was attached to the white subway-tiled walls. There were many silver trays, and machines on stands with wires and tubes. The operating table itself was covered in a large green sheet, onto which two nurses (one male, one female) effortlessly transferred me from the gurney.

The anesthesiologist was already there and waved to me. I saw his eyes smile behind the mask covering his mouth and nose. I could hear my heart beating in my ears. Unlike the television shows that depict rapid heartbeats, I had a slow heartbeat along with low blood pressure. When I looked at the clock, my heartbeat was in tune with the second hand; sixty beats a minute. I closed my eyes and continued the breathing relaxation technique I learned from Dr. Temple.

Dr. Rozbruch arrived within a few minutes and gave me a cheery "good morning" as he proceeded to remove my leg brace.

"What's the marker in your hand for?" I inquired.

"I need to put my signature on your leg and on your belly."

"Really?" I asked, surprised.

"Yup, hospital protocol. In two places. All my work needs to be signed. Two operations for you this morning, so two signatures."

"Will it wash off? Keith will not be happy if he sees you've branded me for life."

And with that short exchange and smiles, everything moved into action. The clock said 8:08, and the date was a fortuitous 8/8.

I don't recall anything past the countdown, as the anesthesia coolly slithered through my body and carried me away. I'm unsure if I imagined Dr. Rozbruch working with masonry tools, or if I dreamed it, or it was actually so and maybe I was watching from above? I never did ask him, but I had been told that, in addition to my own bone from my pelvic girdle or hip, there would also be artificial bone and antibiotics, so maybe the trowel was real.

The next thing I knew, someone was calling my name.

"Elaine, Elaine, wake up." Whomever it was, was gently shaking my hand.

I opened my eyes and was initially confused. "Where am I?"

"You're in the recovery room," said the nurse. "You'll be here for a while, so we can monitor you. Dr. Rozbruch has been to see your husband and will see you later."

"I have a lot of pain," I croaked out, "especially near my hip. Worse than my leg."

"You just had two extensive surgeries according to your chart... Try to wiggle the toes on your feet for me, please."

"Does my husband know where I am? Can he come in to see me? Here?"

"Soon."

"What can you give me for the pain?" I knew I needed something, and the intensity of the pain overrode any thoughts of becoming addicted again. I could not deal with consequences right then.

I ran my tongue around my mouth. "My mouth feels like the Gobi Desert," I complained. "Can I have something to drink?"

"I will bring you some juice. Apple or orange?"

"Apple, please." And then I repeated my plea: "And something for the pain."

"You're already receiving morphine. Once we have monitored you for a while, they will put you on a drip where you can add an additional dose yourself."

I think I gratefully drifted in and out of a light sleep. When I slept, I was not conscious of the pain. I woke to Keith's voice.

"Darling, it's over. Dr. Rozbruch said it all went well. But it will be a few weeks before we will know if it was successful."

"It hurts Keith; it really hurts," I complained. "I think it's just as bad as when they gave me that iodine bath in the trauma hospital, after they stripped me naked."

"I know it was bad. I remember hearing you screaming that night. Now I see they have several ports and tubes. One must be a painkiller. The nurse says you—we—must remain here until they are sure that all your vitals are okay. Then they will move you upstairs."

"Jill? Where is she?"

"Oh, she left after the doctor came to find me and gave us the details. She said she was tired and would call you tomorrow. How lucky you are to have her as a friend (and me too)?"

"And the kids?"

"Phoned them both. Mitch said he would be here tomorrow, and David said he would call you in the morning."

"What time is it?"

"Three."

I must have drifted back off to sleep because the next thing I knew, I woke up in my private hospital room.

My hospital room was on a corner with windows on two sides, overlooking the East River. The sun shining brightly through my massive windows was likely what woke me. The first face I saw, looking intently at me, was my friend and companion, the clock. The large round clock on the wall across from my bed read four. I surmised by the light that it was early evening. I knew I wasn't dreaming.

"Thank you, God," I whispered. "I am happy to be alive, happy to see the sun and feel its warmth, and happy to see Keith." Keith was asleep in a chair beneath the window. I felt a sadness, knowing that it had not been an easy day for him.

I promised God I would think all positive thoughts. I committed myself to asking my brain to send messages to my leg like I did in the trauma hospital. But I directed back to God, *I need your intervention here as well.*

My conversation with God was interrupted by a sharp pain that made me cry out, waking Keith, who ran out of the room. I assumed he went to find a nurse because Hope returned with him. Hope. I loved that I had a nurse with that name!

"Please," I begged, "give me something for the pain. It's incredible."

"You already have a monitored drip. Elaine, for the next twenty-four hours, you'll be able to regulate the dosage you're getting by using this button. If it gets too intense, press the button. Keep the control in your hand. Just know that you can only press at certain intervals and the dosage will only be increased for ten minutes. If you press it before the scheduled interval, it won't react. This is for your safety," she explained.

"On the other side of the bed, I have tied the call button to the side rail. If you need me, it will ring directly on my phone. Now, try to sleep. That will help."

Keith advised me to take the nurse's advice and try to sleep. He said he would use the time to go over to the hotel to get my jacket, and the teddy bear, the clock, and anything else I wanted.

"Can you bring my phone?"

He kissed me on my forehead and both cheeks and reassured me that everything was going to be okay, not to worry. Feeling cared for, I drifted off back to sleep, visiting the land of dreams. I knew that no matter how bad the night ahead would be, it was not the worst night of my life. That prize was still held by April 24th.

Again, the pain woke me. I pressed the ever ready button. It helped. Keith was sitting in the chair next to my bed. According to the clock, an hour had passed. I asked Keith to find the nurse as my stomach was growling, and I thought maybe I could eat something.

Just at that moment, the nurse came in. "Need to check your vitals. How are you doing?"

"Thank God for the magic button," I responded. She smiled. "But I have not had anything to eat."

"Dinner should be up shortly." And then, pulling down my blanket, she said, "I want to just check the incision on your belly. An attending is making rounds and should be here soon."

"And Dr. Rozbruch?" I asked.

"He contacted the nurse's station to say he would be here later and, if you were up, to tell you that he's running behind in surgeries. You must be on his 'A Number One' list." Hope finished examining my incision, and put my gown and blankets back into place.

I think I dropped back to sleep for a bit. Keith was nudging me, letting me know my dinner had arrived.

"Are you okay to eat on your own, or do you want me to help you? While you were asleep, I picked up all the stuff we discussed, as well as having something to eat for myself. How are you?"

"Really? I feel like I've been run over by a Mack truck!"

Keith looked at me with a funny expression. His eyebrows raised, and a smile crinkled his face as he reminded me, "Strange, darling that you would say that. Especially since you were in a car accident! And what, by the way, does it feel like, being run over by a Mack truck?" And we both laughed. Laughing made the pain at the incision on my hip feel worse, but I continued laughing anyway.

"How's my favorite seventy-year-old?" Dr. Rozbruch asked.

"Been better, but I can tell you, been worse too!"

"I'm pleased with the way the surgery went. Now we need to wait."

"How long before I can go home?"

"Well, first you need to get up and trained."

"Trained?"

"Yes, tomorrow we will get you on your leg."

"But..."

"No buts about it! I'll be seeing you in the morning and will take a look at things. Then two of the staff will be here to get you up." When he saw my panicked expression, he went on to explain, "If we want the graft to take, you need to put some weight on your leg."

"No weight or all I have done will be for naught!" I fretted back at the doctor.

"Trust me." He softened his tone. "You need to put at least 25 percent of your weight on that leg. You will have plenty of assistance and support. The staff will show you how to do it. Two people will be here with you. Try the weight, and some prayer, and in two weeks we will know."

"Know what?"

"If the graft has taken." Turning to speak to Keith, he continued, "Don't keep her out too late tonight and no dancing." And with a pat on Keith's shoulder, Dr. Rozbruch left the room.

Keith said he'd stay until I ate but I told him I was tired. I could see the strain and exhaustion on his face too. I told him I was in good hands and if he could just help me with my jacket to reduce the chill I felt and hand me my bear, I was fine for him to go get some rest at the hotel. I checked to make sure I had my cell phone.

The night was long. The hands on the clock moved slower than slow, and I was in constant countdown until I could push the button. I never thought about addiction at all. The nurses, like the last time, were in and out, and getting rest was really challenging. It seemed like every time I could drift off to sleep after pushing the magic button, there they were. Sometimes, it was my body that interrupted what little sleep I could get… pressing the call button for a bedpan, or something to drink other than water, or because I needed to shift my position. Each time I moved, the pain increased.

New York City is so spectacular at night. It was a clear night, and I watched all the lights twinkling right from my bed. I could see the boats on the river. I found the view diverting, but only for short moments of time before the pain would interrupt my pleasure. I repeated to myself the mantra of my physical therapy and the CPM machine days: "No pain, no gain," but it didn't help. Truly, only the magic button helped.

The sun was already up when a doctor (I guessed it was the attending), came to look at my incision and my leg. He introduced himself as Dr. Goldsmith and without pausing, said, "In a little while, once you've eaten your breakfast, we'll be getting you up. Dr. Rozbruch told me to tell you he would be here after lunch." My cell phone rang.

"Sorry, Doc. It's my husband. Only be a few minutes."

Keith said, "I'll be over in five minutes. Anything you want?"

"Yeah. A good cup of coffee would be nice. Stop at Dunkin Donuts. And a muffin, please. Have you told the kids I am okay?"

"Yes, dear." He answered sarcastically as if I was harassing him. *Of course*, he contacted the kids. "I called them again last night."

As he was hanging up, I called out, "Don't go yet." I looked apologetically at Dr. Goldsmith and said, "I don't know about this getting me up, and I'm scared to death. I don't think I can do this without you being here."

"Okay. One stop as per your instructions. I'll be there soon."

Dr. Goldsmith tried to ease my mind. "I have reviewed your chart and I am familiar with your case. Getting you up means getting you off the bed, into the wheelchair, having you get out of the wheelchair and stand up using the walker as an aide. There will be two male nurses in attendance, who will teach you how to take your first steps. It may seem a bit scary—I guess I would be scared too if I were you—but from what Dr. Rozbruch tells me, you have a lot of courage and a great spirit."

CHAPTER 31

ON MY FEET

Several hours later, in marched two young men, one in white scrubs and one in green; one pushing a wheelchair with a bathroom scale occupying the seat, the other carrying phone books and a walker.

"Good morning!" they said in unison. "Are you Miss Elaine?"

"Yes."

"And this man in the chair is?"

"My husband. He came to watch and encourage me. You know, I haven't set my foot on the ground since April 24th, and I'm a little scared. Well, not really… I'm a lot scared."

"My name is Andrew," said the man in the white uniform. "And my partner dressed in green is not Kermit the Frog," he said as he laughed at his own joke. "His name is Kenny. We will be right next to you every step of the way. I promise, we will not let you fall or do anything you should not be doing. Are you ready for your walking lesson?"

"I guess."

"I'll lower the bed, so you can get into the wheelchair by your-self. Can you do that without a slide board?" I nodded in reply and he continued. "Okay then. Once you are seated, I want you to grab onto the walker and pull yourself, or rock yourself, up. And here is what you will do next. I am going to place a telephone book on the floor, close to the bathroom scale. Instead of putting your left foot on the floor, you'll step onto the phone book. Kenny will be on your left, holding you, and you can lean on him for support. I'll be on your right side. You will need to, very gently, put your right foot onto the scale. Merely just touching it. Remember, I will be there holding onto you. Just touch it. You may feel some shocks in your foot. Let me know."

"It has not been on the floor for months," I repeated shakily.

"Think about what you need to do, and why you need to do it. For the graft to take, your leg needs some of your weight. It's like a message going from your foot to your brain."

"Got it." Now he was talking language I understood—messages to the brain.

"And then you will gently push down on the scale until you reach 25 percent of your weight. What do you think you weigh?"

"I guess around 120 pounds."

"Look down when you're doing your gentle push and read the number you see on the scale out loud. Then, if you haven't reached thirty pounds, lift your foot and push a little harder. Once you are around the thirty pounds, then you will need to do that several more times, so you can get a feel of what the pressure on your foot feels like, Okay?

"I guess so."

"We will rest a few minutes; you can sit before you will go through the exercise again." He continued, "If you have some shaking in your arms, this is to be expected. Your body is protecting you by using your arm strength, so you do not injure your leg by putting too much weight on it. Got it?"

"Yeah."

I don't know how to explain the difference between fear and terror. If terror is greater, then I was terrified.

Andrew put non-slip socks on my feet, which he assured me would still let me slide my feet. I eased myself off the bed and onto the wheelchair. The walker and the scale were put in front of me. I rocked myself up and gingerly stepped onto the book. My right leg could not reach the ground due to the height of the book. There was, however, added strain on my arms and left leg. Andrew and Kenny grabbed me around the waist, taking some of the strain and weight off and commanded, "Take your right foot and just place it on the scale. Do not push. Remember, we're holding you. Can you feel the scale?"

"Yes."

"And the sensation in your foot?"

"Well, it feels kind of funny, like just waking up when your foot or leg fell asleep."

"Okay, we'll wait a minute or two. When that feeling stops, push gently down by kind of shifting your weight a little to the right. Look at the screen on the scale and keep leaning, and maybe just a tiny push until it reaches thirty. When it does, shout 'NOW.' Then remove your foot."

I did it. And then they both lowered me down into the wheelchair. Andrew handed me a towel and a glass of orange juice. My arms and legs were shaking. It was hard for me to breathe. The towel was to mop up sweat. I never, ever, sweat. Not even in a sauna. I was starting to understand the difference between fear and terror. The body and brain had taken over.

"Don't try to talk," Kenny said. "In a few minutes, we'll do this again. I assure you; the reaction will not be quite so strong. After a few more times, the fight-or-flight reflex will diminish. Your body will realize it is not in any danger. Then, we start down the hall. Remember, we will be holding onto you. You will not fall, and we'll put the scale in front of you to step on before you take your first few steps."

I looked at the hallway. Like those freaky horror movies or a science fiction dream sequences, the hallway appeared to lengthen and undulate the longer I looked at it.

I suddenly recalled a time in the midst of my divorce, when I was on a beach in East Hampton on a dreary and cold July 4th with my brother, who had kindly brought some Hawaiian Gold pot for me to smoke to alleviate my divorce stress and anxiety.

"It'll make you feel better," he promised. "I'm going to walk on ahead of you. Get up in a few minutes and meet me farther down the beach."

I remember watching him go. He just seemed to get smaller and smaller, and the beach got longer and longer. And the black devils rose up out of the sand, just like at the end of the movie *Ghost*, and started moving towards me—each one of them portraying the fears I was experiencing being a single mom and being on my own after eighteen years of marriage. I was alone and panicked. My brother, who had turned around when he realized I hadn't followed him, found me in the water, walking out to sea. It was the only way I could escape the demons.

I had never experienced that again, until now, when I saw them again. They represented my fears. The fear of never getting out of the chair that had held me captive for the last four months. The fear of always being dependent. The fear of losing my old self forever and, in so doing, the fear of losing Keith.

The voices of my "handlers" brought me back to reality.

"Are you okay? You suddenly went very pale."

Okay Elaine, I bargained with myself, *you can do this. The only way to make those devils go away is to get up and get down the hallway.*

I put my thumb up, signifying yes to my guys. I didn't talk because I thought I might throw up.

Keith never uttered a sound, even though he could see my distress and was probably wondering what I was thinking as I got so pale. He was biting his lip. Maybe terror is contagious?

My break was over. My body and brain needed to be back in the present moment because Andrew said we needed to continue.

Up I went again. They were right there with me and the more times I got up, the more confident I felt. I did finally make it down the hallway, which really was only about ten feet long! I forgot about the pain all during that time. I assume it was diminished due to adrenaline. It's amazing the way the mind can focus intently on one thing and wipe out all other distractions.

Once I got back into the safety of my bed, pain descended on me with a fury. Kenny told me I did great and said he and Andrew would see me later. He told Keith to let me rest, and that Keith looked like he could use some sleep too. And off they went.

Exhaustion overtook me. I woke to the sound of the lunch trays clanging. My table had a note on it from Keith. He had scribbled that he'd be back in a few after getting something to eat and a large coffee.

It was three in the afternoon when Dr. Rozbruch came in.

"The nurses told me you did just fine." He smiled. "The guys will be back just before your dinner and will work with you again. How's the pain?" He leaned over me and checked my leg and the belly incision. "Just to let you know, you are now officially off the magic button. I will leave orders for that IV to be removed. Your pain medicine will be administered orally. I'm leaving orders for one of the staff from customer care to be here in the morning before the nurses come to get you up on your feet, so that arrangements can be made for you to have a therapist come to the house. You need to continue with your walk daily. The other physical therapy as well.

"From what I've been told, for your first time, you've managed quite well. I think if this continues, I can have you get out of here and back home in around two days. Just need to be sure your walking attendant will be there every day.

"I am very proud of you, Elaine," he continued. "What you have been through, well, it hasn't been easy. We need to go day by day; then we will see what your leg looks like." He bent down and gave my hand a little squeeze. "I will see you in about two weeks. Call me anytime with any questions you might have. I'll leave instructions for Rosa to put you through, so long as I am not with a patient. Have a good night."

Two days later I was discharged. The terror had disappeared but not the fears.

CHAPTER 32

HOME AGAIN

110 DAYS SINCE THE ACCIDENT

The routine of my life, once home, fell into the same patterns and schedule as before, except for additional trips to the Long Beach Hospital for physical therapy. At this point, I was able to get on a stationary bicycle and pedal forward. The walks at home, complete with the scale and phone books, were easier and became a bit longer (in both distance and time) each day.

Sean, my walking attendant, as Dr. Rozbruch called him, was a strong young man. Sean could easily have walked right out of the summer pages of an male model calendar! He had a deep tan, dark hair and eyes, lots of muscles, and a cute bum, so I admit, maybe that motivated me a little more to not look too fragile or weak! Sean was entering his final semester towards a Doctor of Physical Therapy degree and told me he hoped to get a position with a physical therapy group in Oceanside, the next town over.

There is much to be said for sleeping in one's own bed, next to the love of my life. Keith continued to wrap his arms around me every night. That helped a lot. I also appreciated not being in a hospital, where sleep was constantly interrupted. A nurse did come to the house every other day to check on me and look at my incisions. As I was up and around at this point, there was no longer a need for daily injections into my belly. I really appreciated the freedom from that, as the incision on my hip was troublesome enough in terms of pain and healing. Even more so than the new staples, which were used to close the incisions in my leg. Maybe, after such a long period, the nerves in my leg had become desensitized?

And most importantly, once I was home, I never touched the oxycodone. At the end of each day, I took a red pen and crossed out the date. Another day of freedom from opioids. The day of knowing I was fully free could not come quickly enough.

CHAPTER 33

WEEK OF AUGUST 20

118 DAYS SINCE THE ACCIDENT

MONDAY, AUGUST 20

I was awakened early Monday, August 20th by several pings in succession from my cell phone. Before I had a chance to review them, the house phone rang. Keith grabbed it. My longtime associate in China, who I called my Chinese brother, was calling me from Hong Kong.

"How's my Jewish sister doing?"

"I'm fine. It's very unusual for you to call me at this time. It's only 6:00 a.m. here. What's up? Problems?"

"Amit sent me an email saying that you are okay and would have the results on Wednesday. And you know what day Wednesday is, don't you?"

"Yeah. It's the day I get the results of my bone graft. Good or bad."

"Don't even think about it. Look at the date. 8/22. How can it not be good? Three lucky numbers!"

I hadn't even thought about it. "Wow" was all I could say.

"Apologize to Keith if I woke him," he said. "Don't forget to email me."

TUESDAY

On Tuesday, there were calls from the children and grandchildren and some of my friends. More positive energy. But somehow, I was not feeling positive. I felt guarded. I had no plan if the bone graft failed.

Keith came home from work early, and as he opened the door, he announced joyously that we should go to the beach, have a drink, and watch the sun go down.

"There's no wind," he said. "It will be just the two of us."

I love that time of day, when the sun is just sinking into the ocean. It was magical. The sky, clouds, and water all shifted colors. We did not speak, we only watched. I will never forget that night, a scene out of a movie, playing in my mind forever.

Keith took my hands in his and said, "Babe, look at me. Can you see in my eyes how deeply I care? How grateful I am to have you and be able to hold you? I fell in love with you, and I am still in love with you. You are my beautiful bride, my life, my partner. Happy camper, that's me. Together, we have the strength to be the happiest, most fulfilled people we can be. After thirty years, now that we are no longer young, please know I have lots and lots of love for my eternal Valentine.

"Knowing you, even with so many people pulling for you and so many prayers coming your way—I know that, you being you,

you can't dismiss the downside of things. I married you for better or worse and if tomorrow is just... well you know what I mean. Remember, Dr. Rozbruch said he would proceed with the bone lengthening thing, which in time, he said would close the holes." He took a couple of deep breaths and then said, "The sun is almost down, a perfect pink-and-blue sky. Time to go."

I looked at that perfect sky and watched most of my fears subside with the setting sun; at least the one about Keith leaving me if I was always to be like I was now.

On the walk back home, Keith pushing me in my chair, he said, "Here's my suggestion about tonight. I went to the butcher and got us a fabulous steak to barbecue. Let's get everything ready for the morning. I'll help you with your shower, then take mine. And after dinner, we should put on a movie and hope we can both get some sleep."

"But," I interrupted him. "What if we don't wake up in time?"

"No worries. I will set three alarms. One on your phone, one on my phone, and one on the clock on the nightstand."

WEDNESDAY

As usual for summertime, there was not a lot of traffic heading into the city.

When we reached the office, the routine was the same as the first visit. Sign in, go down the hall for x-ray. Now that I was used to putting some pressure on my leg, it was not traumatizing. Then an escort brought me to an examination room, where I changed into a pair of paper shorts and sat waiting. The room that day was the same one I had when I first came to see Dr. Rozbruch. I could hear my heart beating in my ears and my hands were ice cold.

191

Although only a few minutes had passed, it seemed like forever. When the door opened, Dr. Rozbruch came in first, followed by Dr. Quig.

"Good morning to you both," Dr. Rozbruch said. "I am going to show you your x-rays." I could tell nothing by looking at his face, or Dr. Quig's either. I took Keith's hand and a deep breath and looked at the screen. Dr. Rozbruch turned to face me. He was smiling.

"You see this white fuzzy here?" he said, pointing. "That's your bone growing."

I started to cry. Was it relief or happiness? It didn't matter. Keith hugged me so hard I nearly lost my breath. Then, he went over to Dr. Rozbruch, saying, "Thank you, thank you."

"I don't know who is more pleased with the result, you or me," laughed Dr. Rozbruch. "Remember, you still have a lot of work to do. You will now have to increase the weight on that leg to 50 percent of your body weight. I am sending an email to Long Beach Hospital's physical therapy department to give you some new exercises. Make an appointment for two weeks from now to take more x-rays and to see me. Do not overdo it. Slowly, slowly. Be sure that you are well balanced before you take your steps with the new weight, and for the first few days, have Keith or your aide beside you, so you can keep checking the scale to be sure that the weight you are pushing down is in the 50 percent range. Not lower, not higher. Call me if you need to. Rosa knows that I am keeping close tabs on you."

He then told me to lay down, so he could check my leg to see if I was still about 90 degrees on the bend. He seemed pleased.

"Dr. Quig will give you another prescription for the PT. You can pick it up at the front desk on your way out. See you in two weeks."

"Keith," I said, "if I could, I would jump up and down for joy. You'll just have to do it for me. I do need a few minutes to compose myself and clean up the mascara from my eyes, so I don't look like a raccoon. Be a dear, and text the kids and the office, and then let's get out of here and go someplace to celebrate!"

The someplace we chose to celebrate was on City Island, New York, where Keith and I had lived for sixteen years, from 1984 to 2000.

City Island, a unique little island off the coast of the Bronx, is just 1.5 miles long and six blocks wide, with a population numbering about 5000. It looks and feels more like Cape Cod than New York City, yet you can get into Manhattan by subway within an hour. On the island, we enjoyed our choice of twenty-seven restaurants, specializing in seafood; five yacht clubs, mainly for sail boaters; an historic nautical museum staffed by volunteers who have lived in City Island all their lives; all surrounded by a variety of adorable shops. The island, near Orchard Beach in the Bronx, is accessible by a small two-lane bridge, or by boat from the start of the Long Island Sound.

City Island held only happy memories for us. When we moved there, we had a brand-new place to live with a newly purchased thirty-one-foot sailboat to go with it, tied to a mooring less than 300 feet from our unit. The boat was christened *Joint Venture II*, recognizable to the local sailing community by a red, white, and blue jib sail and crossed American and British flags on the stern.

Our residential unit was two levels, with 96" quarter circle windows on the second floor that looked out on the water, and a working fireplace in the living room. Very, very romantic. With all our good memories and the vacation feel of City Island, it was fitting for us to spend our celebration day there.

Keith had a hard time forgiving me for giving up that condo, moving off the small island and out to Long Island. My accountant business brain calculated that we needed to purchase a London apartment as our new office at Heathrow was growing by leaps and bounds, so having three mortgages was more than we could afford... New York, Miami, and London. We had to give one up. After 9/11, we agreed that it was actually good that we were out on Long Island.

Our favorite restaurant on City Island was the Original Crab Shanty. Joe, the owner, was a good friend of ours. Keith called ahead, spoke to Joe, asking him to put a bottle of champagne on ice and advising him that we would be there in about thirty minutes.

"What's the occasion, Brit?" Joe asked.

"We are celebrating the start of the bone growth of Elaine's shattered leg," Keith answered.

Joe surprised us. "In that case, the champagne is on me. I am thrilled for both of you! Always glad to see you guys."

It was a perfect afternoon, just the two of us. As much as we knew our friends and family wanted to celebrate with us, we needed this time to ourselves. The months since the accident had been filled with uncertainty and fear. Now that was all behind us. It wasn't only the beginning of the healing of my leg, but also the healing of our individual spirits.

THURSDAY

The following day, I set a schedule with Keith so he could position me to get accustomed to the pressure of the scale and be there for the first few days that I was walking using 50 percent of my weight on my injured leg.

Walking was not "walking" in a true sense. I would rock back and forth using only my left leg, holding onto the walker, until I could stand up, and then measure 50 percent on the scale. The books and the scale were always in the same spot in my bedroom, and once I was confident, I would set off. My arms on the walker, and my left foot was used to move me forward. To take the next step, I had to push the walker forward, make a little hop, and slide with my left foot forward, put my right foot down, and then get my right foot to slide up even to the left leg. It was not easy and very tiring. I concentrated on not losing my balance. I always had Keith and my aide on either side.

Physical therapy was three times a week, with lots of exercises to do at home. I remained diligent when it came to this. My friend, the clock, with its alarm at my beck and call, was always there to help. It was set to time the walk, the home exercises, and to remind me to be ready for Keith to take me to the hospital for therapy. I still used the slide board for most of my transitions into and out of the wheelchair.

Besides taking me to the beach, sometimes Keith would wheel me all the way to the grocery store, about three blocks from home. Sitting outside, I would converse with whomever happened to stop by and ask me, "What happened to you? Are you okay to be out here alone?"

I would always respond, "I'm fine. My husband is doing the shopping and I am the cart to carry the groceries home." There were always smiles when I said this.

CHAPTER 34

KEEP UP THE GOOD WORK

132 DAYS SINCE THE ACCIDENT

Two weeks later, I was on my way to see Dr. Rozbruch once again. In the examination room, once new x-rays had been taken, I was very nervous.

"Keith, what if there is still no improvement? Have you thought about how life would continue for us? How will I be able to work? I'll never be able to get up all of those stairs."

Keith interrupted me. "Well, darling, you will just have to walk up on your hands," he said, smiling. "Of course, you can work. We'll have your office brought home to Long Beach. I am looking into renting a small studio apartment in a building with an elevator. But stop jumping the gun. Let's see what Dr. Rozbruch has to say." Just at that moment, the door opened and in the handsome doctor walked. Smiling.

"Your x-rays show an improvement in the bone growth. Elaine, I am so pleased. So, now, onward and upward. Continue what you are doing and increase the weight. Go to 75 percent, but be careful not to put all of your weight on that leg. And be back here in another three weeks, so we can check the progress. Continue the same exercises with the physical therapists, and don't forget to do all of your home exercises too."

He then turned to Keith and said, "Before I get on with the rest of my day, I need to hug your wife. Looking at her x-rays made my day. Maybe even my week. Take good care of her. She has an indomitable spirit and a tremendous support system in you. Keep up the good work. That's my message to you both."

CHAPTER 35

OCTOBER

156 DAYS SINCE THE ACCIDENT

Seven weeks after the bone graft operation, the bone was 80 percent healed. Smiling, Dr. Rozbruch said to me, "Okay, Miss Miracle, you can now stand up with your full weight on both legs and practice walking with a walker. Best to do this only when Keith or your aide or someone else is alongside you, in case you lose your balance. Physical therapy needs to continue two to three times a week for now, and you need to do all of your home exercise on the days that you don't have physical therapy. Be back here in a month, so I can analyze your progress." Then he gave me a big hug. "Keep up the good work."

As soon as I got home, Keith, at my insistence, got me the walker.

"Okay," I said to him, "show me how you walk."

"You're joking, right?"

"No. Do you start with your left foot or your right foot? And do you walk heel first or toe first? Walking is putting one foot in front of the other, right? How far in front? I only shuffle now, so show me."

It took about two weeks of practice and concentration, and a lot of talking to myself, before I didn't have to think about what to do with my legs and feet. The steps were small. The left foot had a longer stride than the right foot. I am not sure why or how, but eventually my brain sent the correct commands.

All of my right shoes now required a heel lift, as my right leg was a little over half an inch shorter than my left. Sneakers were best for walking, still are. Any other flat shoes had to have rubber soles to prevent slipping. I walked only slowly. But I actually did walk. After a time, I was able to migrate away from the walker and just use a cane. And always, always very carefully.

CHAPTER 36

BACK IN THE T-BIRD

5 MONTHS SINCE THE ACCIDENT

Early one Sunday morning at the end of September, Keith shocked me by saying, "It's time you got behind the wheel of your car."

"No. Absolutely not," I protested.

"Yes, it's time, and the time is today. The beaches are closed, and the parking lots will be empty. I'll drive you there and you can just see how it feels."

My car, a 2002 Thunderbird, sits very low to the ground. Even with how well my legs had healed, getting into the passenger side still took a bit of doing. Once we arrived at the empty parking lot, it took an extra effort to get in on the driver's side because of the steering wheel.

"How do you feel?" Keith asked. "Comfy? Okay, put the key into the ignition, foot on the brake, and start the car. Do not touch the gear shift. All I want you to do is gently press down on the gas and then the brake. The car is in park, and you are not going anywhere.

Get a feel for the pedals. Be sure to keep your hands on the wheel. You'll know by the sound of the engine if you are pressing too hard on the accelerator. Gently, very gently, then move off the accelerator onto the brake. When you feel you are ready, shut the car off."

I followed all his instructions, and then I shut the engine off.

We started again.

"Put your foot on the brake. I'll move the gear shift in the center console into first gear. When you take your foot off the brake, only rest it on the accelerator; don't press it. The car will move forward but not a lot, and then you can give it a little gas. Not to worry, you will not go faster than fifteen mph. Be gentle on the gas, be gentle on the brake, and make sure you use the brake to come to a full stop before you go back to putting your foot on the accelerator. Repeat on the gas, and repeat on the brake, and now drive around the perimeter of the parking lot."

I had flashbacks to the days when I learned to drive a car for the first time. My father taught me how to drive in the supermarket parking lot, on Sundays when the store was closed.

My perception was that I was going a lot faster than I was. After the first few minutes, I was no longer feeling afraid, but exhilarated. I was really proud of myself. Halfway round the lot, I told Keith I needed to stop. I couldn't believe how tired I felt.

"Stop and I will put the car into park; you can shut off the engine," he responded. "We'll put the top down and enjoy the sunshine. Are you comfortable with what you've done? Were you scared?"

"At first a little, and then apprehensive. Remember, this car and I have been together over ten years. It is almost like a part of me."

That was lesson number one. Each subsequent practice was better than the one before. I was soon able to increase my speed to 30 mph—in second gear only. When I told Keith I was ready, he let me put the car in drive. I got up to 40 mph too quickly and was a bit unnerved.

Keith said, "Ease off the gas, and gently put your foot on the brake to stop the car. Put the car in park and shut it off. When you're ready to try again, we'll practice in reverse and you can try back parking using the lines on the spaces."

I appreciated Keith's patience and told him so.

With each practice, my confidence increased. Eventually, I started to drive on the local streets, but not during high traffic times.

As happy as Keith professed to be for my progress, there were times I could see a funny look on his face. Not really sadness, but close to that. My dependence on him was decreasing daily. All my life, I have been very capable and in-charge. People (especially men, going back to cave-man times) feel fulfilled by being needed. Keith probably felt good that he could be there for me and provide support. Maybe, like a mother who sees the increasing independence of her child, there is a certain sadness that comes with the realization that the bonding that comes with that dependency will never be repeated.

CHAPTER 37

THE REST OF MY LIFE BEGINS

For a long time, I continued to carry a cane, even though I did not need it. Anytime I knew I would be going into crowds, I took it because it acted as a deterrent, keeping, people (especially children) away from me. When I walk now, as then, I scan the ground in front of me to be sure that there is nothing that could get me into trouble.

When I am driving and need to change lanes, I have to be sure that I have plenty of space to move over, and that no car behind me is approaching quickly. I feel most vulnerable if I cannot get over in time to get off on my exit. In that situation, I will go past my exit and backtrack to where I need to go.

Stairs are still problematic. Up, not so much. If I were to lose my balance and fall going up, I believe I would not fall down too far. Of course, I could get banged up a bit. Going down, well that's another story. It is not that I can't do it; it's the fear of tumbling and not being able to stop. I hold the bannister, then lower my right foot onto the step below, and then bring my left foot down beside it. Just the way they showed me in rehab.

Every three months, I made visits to see Dr. Rozbruch. In August of 2014, two years almost to the day from Dr. Rozbruch's first surgery on me, he removed the plate from my leg. He explained that eventually the bone would start to grow over the plate and if, or when, I needed a knee replacement, it would not be possible.

There were marks like tiny circles of rust where the screws had been. It took almost a year for them to disappear. And after what I had been through, this surgery was a piece of cake. Although the x-rays showed that I had bone on bone in my knee joint, there was very little pain, so I ignored any thought of another surgery.

However, by August 2016, I changed my mind. I still had hardly any pain. What pushed me to do it was not my advancing age, although age was a factor.

On Christmas Day, 2015, Keith was diagnosed with AML (Acute Myeloid Leukemia), a fast-advancing blood cancer with no cure. I wanted to be fully able to be there for my husband.

After Keith's diagnosis, I sold our apartment on Long Island at the end of September, and the house in Hollywood, Florida, shortly thereafter. There was no time to do any packing on my own, or any unpacking due to the quick sale of both. Paid people went in and got done what needed to be done. All the contents of the homes went into storage. My priority was Keith.

My husband and I moved into a furnished apartment in New York City, close to the hospital that was treating his cancer where, thank goodness, Keith was responding well to the treatments.

When transfusions and chemotherapy started to improve his blood components, I elected to start my own physical therapy to strengthen my muscles, hoping that I could go ahead with the knee replacement. The timing of the knee replacement was perfect. Keith's blood stabilized for about eight months, giving us some quality time together and time to plan before his levels started dropping again as the cancer advanced.

Cancer won the battle and the war. Keith passed away in October of 2017, defying the odds on the length of life after diagnosis. I know for certain each day I live becomes more precious; family and friends are dearer.

It is in the fall, around the anniversary of Keith's death, and especially on the anniversary date of the accident in April, that I find myself reflecting on what I have accomplished. I do not run, skip, hop, or jump, but I walk in much the same way I did before the accident. And I can dance too, sometimes even in high heels. But not for long (more due to asthma than fatigue).

A good friend of mine, Rabbi Zurchind, explains my journey in this way: He says many times, what we experience has been predestined—predetermined. It happens when it needs to happen. And the lessons learned are not only what we ourselves learn, but what we teach to others. Not directly, but indirectly. What others witnessed by looking at you, watching your reactions and relating to what they saw, becomes instrumental in changing their lives, maybe more than changing yours. Rabbi Zurchind reminded me that many people have said to me that they would not have had the courage to do what we can call "x," without seeing how I handled myself, especially in those first few months.

On my final visit to Dr. Rozbruch, he asked me if I would write about my journey. He said, "Elaine, I think it will inspire my patients (especially the older ones) to never give up."

If my story can help other people face their own hardships and challenges to know that survival and thriving again is possible, then I have made a difference.

CHAPTER 38

FLORIDA:
A NEW BEGINNING

I moved to Florida permanently in November of 2017, having driven down from New York, accompanied by my son, Mitch. My other son, David, had taken over the family business and I was, for the most part, retired. New home, new life. This was the first time in my life I would be living alone.

Mitch and I exchanged awkward, curbside, never-want-to-let-you-go hugs at the airport in Palm Beach as he had to get back to New York and his family. I was sad to see him go. We had a great trip down and got to talk about things more deeply than we normally managed with quick phone calls.

Thirty minutes later, with the assistance of my GPS, I arrived at my new home. To say I was horrified when I open opened the front door does not even begin to describe what ran through my mind, or my body's reaction to what I saw.

There were boxes piled upon boxes. Boxes on top of the furniture. Furniture on top of furniture. Furniture on top of boxes.

The screened-in patio area was piled high with all the outdoor furniture from both houses. The grill was not stacked but was leaning precariously to one side and seemed one breeze away from tipping over.

Two movers had combined two houses into one space. And more than the clutter, I had no way to understand what was in any of the boxes. The local mover had used a colored tape, which at least differentiated Florida boxes from New York boxes. There was barely enough space on the floor to navigate from one side of the room to the other.

Thankfully, the movers left one of the bathrooms and half the bed in the master bedroom clear of boxes. The guest bedroom set had been assembled, and only half that mattress had boxes on it too.

I had the option of going to a hotel but decided that it was better to wake up and just attack the mess in the morning. If I found a comfortable place to stay, I might not come back!

I closed the front door, leaving a light on in the house and one light on outside, so I would not damage myself on the way back in the dark. I'd decided to get something to eat and pick up a few bottles of vodka to ease the pain of having to return to the huge, overwhelming job ahead of me.

Anything I might have needed just for the night was in a box somewhere, and I did not know where to even begin to find such items. Bed Bath and Beyond, located in the same shopping center as the restaurant, came to the rescue. I purchased linens, a pillow, a coffee pot, some hand soap for the bathroom, and two towels. I picked out some plastic dishes, cups, and tableware. Dinner was unhurried, as the longer I stayed away, the better. It was getting late and it was a weekday night, so I left the restaurant when I realized I was the only person remaining.

Gritting my teeth, I entered the house again and managed to clear a pathway to the guest bedroom. I dropped my BB&B bags on the clear side of the bed, brought my suitcases in from the car, made the bed, plugged in my computer, drank some vodka, and eventually fell asleep—only to be awakened by a really noisy bird at 6:00 a.m. Welcome to Florida!

Making my way through the forest of boxes with the coffee pot and coffee, I saw one of the drawers directly under the cooktop was open. I closed it.

I had no toilet paper, but I did have tissues. In retrospect, perhaps TP should have been something I added to my list of items at BB&B!? A shower made me feel better. At least there was hot water and air conditioning, and electricity to charge my computer and cell phone. I tried to imagine where to begin but could not. Vanese, my housekeeper for eighteen years at the Hollywood house, was coming to assist and could make that decision.

Morning coffee is a magic potion. It sets the world to right, gives us energy and a feeling of strength and well-being. I was now ready to face the garage. If I could make space in the garage, then I could bring what I didn't need in the house out there, and work on those items later.

Big mistake. The car carrier was due to arrive in two days, bringing my T-Bird and the Maserati. Three cars and nowhere to put them. I was sure the homeowner's association would fine me for parking my car in the driveway or street overnight. That was the least of my worries.

Back in the kitchen, I plugged in the washed coffee pot to make another batch of energy… and when I walked past the stove, that same drawer was open again. My thought was that one of the movers had put something in it, and maybe it was unbalanced? It was empty, except for a few dead bugs. Yuck.

I stripped the bed I had slept in and placed the bedding in the bathtub so as not to interfere with the unpacking. I needed the bed space to lay out items as they came out of the cartons in that room.

At least the movers had hung all the clothes in the closets, and it looked like they had separated mine from my husband's.

My house phone rang a few minutes after 9. It was the gatehouse advising me that Vanese had arrived.

"Door's open," I shouted when I heard her knock. Vanese, a tall, strong, highly-efficient woman, entered the room smelling like clean air and greeted me with a warm hug.

"I'm so sorry," she whispered into my neck. There were tears in her brown eyes. Vanese had adored my husband. She flipped over his English accent.

"There's coffee in the pot," I said, "and some plastic cups. I have some sugar I confiscated from Dunkin' Donuts, but no milk or cream."

"No matter, Miss Em." (She had always called me Miss Em.) "Well," she said, looking around, "hopefully the movers had the good sense to label the boxes, so let's look for ones that we can unpack quickly that might say 'kitchen' or 'bathroom'. At least we can find some dishes and some pots, and maybe some sheets and towels too.

"But first, I'm going to clear a pathway between the center island sink and the stove. I'm going to need the sink for water, and if we find the box with whatever was under the sink in the old house, I can put it away straightaway."

Unlike my previous homes, this new house had an open-concept design where the kitchen, dining room, and living room are all in one space. No walls. There is a center island that creates a separation between the kitchen and dining room. The cabinets and appliances are set up in an L shape, which separates the living room area from the other areas. Bedrooms and bathrooms are at either end.

As Vanese walked around the center island, she looked at me and said, "Miss Em, what's this drawer doing open?"

"I don't know. It was open last night. I closed it and found it open again this morning, and closed it then too."

Looking straight at me, she said, "I bet it's Mister Keith coming to say hello."

"No, no. I think there must be something wrong with the balance. Once we can fill it with some stuff, then it won't open." I was thinking, there's a logical explanation for everything, right?

"Okay," she said, "have it your way. But I know better. He loves you so much, he needs to let you know he's here to protect you, and this way he is letting you know he is still here, even though you can't see him or hear him."

"Well not unless the drawer has a squeak," I said, smiling at my own joke about "hearing" him.

We proceeded to open the boxes marked "kitchen" first, and I put some trivets and pots I would not need into the mysterious drawer, hoping that my arrangement would put the drawer in perfect balance.

The drawer opened twice more that day. Each time, I readjusted the items, taking out some and putting others in. I also filled the bottom drawer with things that weighed more and were not needed for every day. Maybe the bottom drawer was somehow connected to the upper one, I pondered.

Each time the drawer opened, Vanese repeated herself, attributing the opening of the drawer to Keith. Each time I poo-pooed it. Vanese's logic was that "He's only been gone three weeks. He's still in the world of in-between. And he wants to make sure you are okay."

On her way out, she reminded me, "I need to clean Miss Bea's [one of my local friends] house tomorrow, so I'll be back in two days. You try to get some rest."

My first night on my own in the new house, the vodka, after a long drive, had done its job. Sleep had come easily. Night two, restless after thirty minutes in the bed, I got up deciding that if I had a drink (maybe a brandy), I could read and then get to sleep. As I walked between the two hall closet doors, I felt compelled to open the one that held Keith's clothing. The smell of his cologne still lingered. Without thinking about it, I buried my face in his clothes and prayed that the salt in the tears I was shedding would help to heal the ache in my chest.

The next morning the mystery kitchen drawer was closed. I said to myself, *See, you have finally got the right balance.*

After my coffee, when I opened the front door, right in front of me on the doormat was a perfect, large, spotless white feather. *How curious*, I thought. Something inside of me said, *Don't put it in the garbage. Keep it.* I thought, *I'll put it in a plastic bag on top of the washing machine so I can remember where it is and then it won't get tossed out with packing material from all the boxes.*

I continued on my own for the rest of the day, emptying boxes until the cars arrived. They were being delivered by a professional auto moving company. The cars arrived on a multi-car monster of a truck. I instructed the driver to put one car on the street, and the other to pull into the driveway. My car was already in the garage. I'd worry about the potential fine situation later.

The phone rang just as I walked back into the house. It was my friend Bea calling to see how I was getting on. I didn't tell her about the drawer, but I shared my morning news about the feather on the door mat.

"You know about white feathers, don't you?" Bea asked excitedly.

I responded, laughing, "They come from birds."

"No, dear. If you find a white feather, it means that an angel came to visit. It's a gift to remind you to take care of yourself, that you shouldn't get stressed, to calm down. White feathers appear when angels are near. Maybe it's Keith. Maybe not. Maybe you have your own special angel just saying hello."

"Great, Bea. Just what I needed to hear. It's still early evening and I am well past the age of bedtime stories!"

"Believe what you want. Any other things happening out of the ordinary?" she asked.

"Yeah. I have a drawer that keeps opening in the kitchen. Must be out of balance. But it's stopped now. I think I was finally able to position some pots in just the right spaces to create balance."

My friend continued, "Don't be surprised if it continues to open. But eventually it will stop. You'll see."

"Just to let you know," I said, "I have read that sometimes, after a loved one has died, that there are signs that the loved one is still near. Things like butterflies that keep flying around, a certain smell like someone's perfume, the sight of a red cardinal, lights that go off and on for no reason, dreams of that person but not, I repeat *not*, drawers opening!"

"Well, your husband loved to cook. Maybe his spirit has taken up domicile in your kitchen?"

I refrained from telling her that she was ridiculous and just said good night. I wondered if Vanese had told Bea my story and given rise to these theories about Keith and the drawer?

Several times a week, the drawer continued to open for no apparent reason, occasionally startling me. If I was in front of the stove, the drawer would hit me when it opened. No amount of arranging or rearranging helped. Sometimes, it would happen when a friend came to visit, and always when Vanese came to clean. She'd just tell me when it happened and show me the drawer. I gave up. I decided to accept what she told me.

As for the white feathers, two more appeared out of nowhere. The first one appeared right inside the house, close to my bed, when I came home after being away for Christmas for nearly two weeks.

After a truck had come to pick up the Cadillac CTS and Maserati I had sold, another feather was found in the garage under where the Maserati had been parked.

I am not sure what my friends thought when I told them about the mystical drawer. The drawer still opened on its own, but less frequently now. Even a few friends had seen it open when they were visiting. Sometimes, when I was alone and it happened, after I closed it and it reopened, I took to scolding Keith... well not really scolding but compelling him to stop.

T-Bird Sweet Sixteen

In May, when there were no more boxes and the garage was emptied of excess cars, I decided to have some friends come to my home. The occasion was to celebrate my T-Bird's Sweet Sixteen. The car was festooned with pink ribbons and balloons in the garage, with a big sign on the hood saying *Happy Birthday Sweet Sixteen*. The house was decorated all in pink, with balloons and pink flowers, and a pink cake that had a picture of my T-Bird on it. There was plenty of pink champagne to drink too.

On the night of my party, a good friend of Keith's (originally from New York and now living in Florida), with his wife, were invitees. Eddie and I were in the kitchen talking about old times and how much he missed Keith. Eddie was facing me, leaning against the stove, and I was just opposite him. When the drawer hit him in the rear end, he jumped.

I said "Eddie, that's Keith."

"Listen, Elaine… it can't be."

"Eddie," I said, "trust me, it's him." And then the drawer performed for Eddie by opening twice more, one after the other, when he had closed it.

I needed to keep the belief going that it really was Keith. It helped with the grief and loneliness, and the days I called *bad heart days*. BHD are the days when you get that pain in your chest. Sometimes when the pain came, the drawer would open, sometimes not. As the time between openings stretched further apart, I took to taking out my phone and taking a photo of the open drawer. The photos were date and time stamped. One of the last times the drawer opened was August 4, 2019.

As the months went on and the opening trick had completely stopped, I consoled myself that Keith knew I was okay and that everything I needed to do as result of his death was taken care of. I often thought that perhaps the drawer was not only to console me and make me believe he was still watching over me, but maybe he needed to see me, so he wouldn't feel so bad about us being separated.

At some point, after I joined a writing work group, I thought about my Keith drawer and decided it was a good topic for a short story. I felt that the whole thing was really quite extraordinary. I titled the story *The Opening Drawer*. It would be up to the reader to believe it as truth or not.

I use my dining room table as a desk, and this is where I was when I began to write on Monday, June 1st, 2020. It was 11:28 a.m. when I rose up to get another cup of coffee from the kitchen area. From where I sit at the table, I can only see the top of the stove. Looking over the stove from a standing position, I saw the drawer was open. It freaked me out. My hands started to shake, and I really thought I was going to faint.

I called my friend Jill, because I knew she would be able to help calm me down. She still lived in New York. I grabbed my phone but before I dialed, I snapped a picture. The question that tickled my brain was *why now?* It had been a long time from August 4th, 2019 to June 1st, 2020. Was it because I was writing the story?

Jill reminded me of something I had incorporated into Keith's eulogy.

"'Love beyond the world cannot be separated by it.' Keith's just letting you know he is still close and watching over you," she concluded.

It took me several weeks to understand why the drawer opened on the 1st, and again on the 10th in the beginning of June, whereas it had not since August 4th of 2019. I had, in those two plus years I'd been in this house, made a life for myself. I had gained strength and had lost my fear of being alone.

Keith's task on this earth, I believe, was to keep me safe and protect me. The drawer openings happened around the time Florida was experiencing a dramatic increase in the number of positive tests and deaths due to the Coronavirus. Florida was the new hot spot. I feel in my heart and soul this was Keith's way to notify me that I was not alone and would never be alone. He was still looking out for me, and I should know I was protected. The fact that the drawer opened twice was meant to reinforce the message. It was him saying, "I love you and I am here for you always."

9 781951 591632